Praise for

HEALTHY TO 100

"The right book at the right time. *Healthy to 100* is a fascinating and hopeful voyage through five of the world's healthiest and longest-lived countries, revealing how those societies are supporting connection, community, and purpose—and healthier, longer life as a result. Ken Stern weaves together the latest research with his own keen eye for story and detail in this compelling and fun read. For anyone thinking about what the second half of life should look like, *Healthy to 100* is a must-read."

—Chip Conley, *New York Times* bestselling
author of *Learning to Love Midlife*

"Rather than learn from forty-year-old tech bros advocating unproven supplements and radical exercise programs, Ken Stern goes around the world to gather wisdom from the everyday lives of older people to find what makes for a healthy, engaged, and purposeful life wherever you live. Success lies less in cracking human biology and more in cracking human connectivity. An insightful and entertaining book that is a must-read for anyone who is thinking about how to live a longer, healthier life."

—Andrew Scott, coauthor of *The 100-Year Life*

"In the spirit of E. M. Forster's famous mandate, 'Only Connect,' Ken Stern's *Healthy to 100* reveals social connection to be the key to long, healthy, and joyous lives. *Healthy to 100* takes us on a journey from the dusty streets of Presidio, Texas, to the futuristic towers of Singapore, crisscrossing the globe to illuminate the power of social health and intergenerational ties. Beautifully written, filled with indelible stories, and deeply rooted in research, Stern's book offers our best blueprint for realizing the vast promise of the longevity revolution, as individuals and as societies."

—Marc Freedman, author of *How to Live Forever*

"Which country has unlocked the secret to aging well? After traveling the globe to study the world's longest-lived populations, Ken Stern discovered something surprising: it's not Mediterranean diets, cutting-edge healthcare, or exercise regimens that matter most. The real key to a long, vibrant life lies in our connections with one another. *Healthy to 100* is both a wake-up call about our loneliness epidemic and a hopeful roadmap for building the social infrastructure we need to thrive at every stage of life. Compassionate, insightful, and surprisingly uplifting, this book will change how you think about growing older—and inspire you to invest in what truly matters."

—Laura L. Carstensen, founding director,
Stanford Center on Longevity

HEALTHY
TO 100

ALSO BY KEN STERN

*Republican Like Me: How I Left the Liberal
Bubble and Learned to Love the Right*

*With Charity for All: Why Charities Are
Failing and a Better Way to Give*

HEALTHY TO 100

HOW STRONG SOCIAL TIES
LEAD TO LONG LIVES

KEN STERN

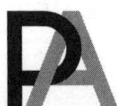

PA

PUBLICAFFAIRS

New York

PublicAffairs
Hachette Book Group
1290 Avenue of the Americas, New York, NY 10104
www.publicaffairsbooks.com
@Public_Affairs

Printed in the United States of America

First Edition: October 2025

Published by PublicAffairs, an imprint of Hachette Book Group, Inc. The Public-
Affairs name and logo is a registered trademark of the Hachette Book Group.

The Hachette Speakers Bureau provides a wide range of authors for speaking events.
To find out more, go to hachettespeakersbureau.com or email
HachetteSpeakers@hbgusa.com.

PublicAffairs books may be purchased in bulk for business, educational, or
promotional use. For more information, please contact your local bookseller or the
Hachette Book Group Special Markets Department at special.markets@hbgusa.com.

The publisher is not responsible for websites (or their content) that are not owned by
the publisher.

Library of Congress Control Number: 2025003604

ISBNs: 9781541705012 (hardcover), 9781541705036 (ebook)

LSC-C

Printing 1, 2025

For Nate, may he live healthy to 100

CONTENTS

Introduction

MIYAKO CLAPS HER hands in delight and flies past us, her sandals clacking rhythmically as she runs toward the bridge. She reaches the other end and turns back to look at us, as though in wonder that we haven't kept pace. Hiro shoots me a sideways look, a combination of amusement and amazement, because it's not every day that you get left in the dust by an eighty-eight-year-old woman.

It wasn't a total surprise to us, though. We had traveled that morning to the rural city of Ukiha, about two hours east of Fukuoka in southern Japan, to visit the offices of Ukiha no Takara Co., Ltd., a small food services company specializing in traditional Japanese foods. The company has achieved a modest public recognition for its unusual hiring strategy, as it principally employs women over the age of sixty: Those over the age of seventy-five are called "grand-mothers," and those between the ages of sixty and seventy-five are labeled "grandmother juniors." It is an unusual hiring strategy to say the least, reflecting the owner's desire to engage the elders of his community, but it also makes a certain amount of sense from a human resources perspective in a country where 30 percent of the population is over sixty-five and the majority of that group wants to keep working.

On the train out to Ukiha, Hiro, a Japanese journalist who had signed on as my translator, and I strategized about the interviews.

We had plenty of time, since Ukiha doesn't sit on any of the main train lines and is only served by creaky commuter trains rather than the Shinkansen (bullet trains) for which Japan is justifiably famous. We chugged out of Fukuoka on one train, only to change at a small station where a row of commuter bicycles sat unlocked, unwatched, and untroubled. Our second train eventually deposited us in Ukiha, a town of twenty-seven thousand sometimes called the "Kingdom of Fruits" in recognition of its agricultural traditions.

We were scheduled to talk with three of the grandmothers, ranging in age from seventy-seven to eighty-eight, and I was a little concerned about the conditions of the interview: Would the grand-mothers have the energy for a long conversation, would they be comfortable talking with us, and would they be interested in the topic that I wanted to explore with them—the relationships between work, social connection, and health?

I needn't have worried. Our interview takes place in the cramped kitchen, an enormous pot of potatoes gently bubbling in the background. There are no chairs, and it is hot and crowded, but it quickly becomes quite clear that Hiro and I will tire before the grandmothers. Miyako, Keiko (age eighty-two), and Sakie (age seventy-seven) are full of energy and life, laughing and clap-ping at each other's answers and enjoying the novelty of a visitor from afar.

Miyako was born in Ukiha and met her husband there but spent most of her life as a Kyoto housewife. After her husband's retirement, they returned to their hometown. With her children and grandchildren grown and distant, Miyako became bored and lonely, and felt that she lacked purpose in life. She saw her friends taking jobs, so Miyako entered the workforce for the first time, joining some of her contemporaries three mornings a week in the Ukiha no Takara company kitchen. It's an act of courage, the willingness to try such new things so late in life, but it's one, Miyako assures me, that has been amply rewarded. "I love coming to work, being with my friends. It gives me purpose and meaning to my life that would not otherwise be there." She credits getting out of the house and joining her friends at work for her remarkable health and energy, and for saving her from a life of isolation and loneliness.

Ukiha no Takara roughly translates as "Ukiha miracle," and it is tempting to view the boundless energy and joy of the grandmothers as just a little short of miraculous. But I start with this story for precisely the opposite reason, because Miyako's story is neither particularly miraculous from a health perspective nor even unusual in Japan. Japan has the longest life expectancy of any country in the world, and more importantly, it has the longest *healthy* life expectancy, the number of years a person can expect to live disability-free and in good health. The average Japanese person can now expect to live over seventy-four years in good health—four years longer than in the United Kingdom and *eight* years longer than in the United States.[1]

Japan is also the country in which the highest percentage of people over sixty-five continue to work; roughly 25 percent of the people over sixty-five are active members of the labor force.[2] That number is double that of the UK and three times the rate in Germany by comparison. And people across Japan will tell you that the high employment figures and the strong health data are closely related. When I ask Miyako, Keiko, and Sakie whether working has contributed to their remarkable good health, they all laugh like I just cracked a good joke, because for them, and for most Japanese, it is self-evident that the social connection and purpose that come with work are critical contributors to their vitality and good health.

———

In 1938, in the depths of the Depression, researchers at Harvard launched an ambitious study to identify the sources of happiness and health, to understand what makes some people thrive and others struggle. The study, which eventually became known as the Harvard Study of Adult Development, started with two distinct groups. The researchers first enrolled 268 Harvard sophomores. These were presumed to be the leaders of tomorrow—and indeed the group included John F. Kennedy and Ben Bradlee, the legendary editor of *The Washington Post* during the Watergate era—though the researchers were careful to ensure that the study group balanced scholarship students with the scions of the Brahmin families of Boston. The Harvard group was supplemented with 456 boys who came from some of Boston's most troubled and disadvantaged neighborhoods. These boys were mostly the children of immigrants and were typically saddled with a combination of poverty and limited educational and social opportunity, which stood in sharp contrast to the seemingly boundless opportunity unfolding before the Harvard students.

The researchers had the extraordinarily ambitious agenda of following these 724 men across their lifetimes, through war and migration, marriage and divorce, work and unemployment, and in some cases incarceration, and yet the original founders of the study would have been astonished to see what has happened. Not only did the Harvard team and its successors (which is now in its fourth generation of researchers) successfully follow this group, it ultimately expanded the study group to include some 1,300 spouses and descendants. Closing in on its ninth decade, the Harvard Study of Adult Development is now the longest-running longitudinal health study in American history. It is extraordinary not only in its longevity but in its comprehensiveness.[3] Every year, the researchers collect a treasure trove of data on each participant. Health data of course including blood draws, DNA samples, EKG reports, brain scans, and (in the early days) phrenology studies of the shape and weight of skulls. But that's just a part of it: They also log employment data; voting records; behavioral information such as smoking and drinking; and the results of extensive biennial interviews with participants, their spouses, and their children.

It is a study that is unprecedented in scope and detail, and what the researchers have found is startling, both in its conclusion and in its clarity. After parsing through eighty-five years of data, the researchers have concluded that there is a formula for a healthy life. It's not weight, exercise levels, the quality of diet, or even income that most impacts healthy longevity. It is the quality of relationships, the social fitness, you might say, of the people involved. It's really an astounding thing. We've been conditioned to judge our health by a scorecard of numbers: our weight, our blood pressure, our cholesterol level, our caloric intake. But none of that matters as much as our relationships. It all boils down to the idea—as Robert Waldinger, the current director, has said—of "being engaged in activities I care about with people I care about." If you want to come up with the recipe for successful aging, you need to start with the key ingredient, and that is the nature of your relationships and your social connections. If you want to know how to live a healthy and rewarding life, you start with *social health.*

You may not be shocked by the idea that social health is important to your well-being and that, conversely, loneliness is a danger to your health. After all, the UK in 2018 created the position of minister of loneliness, a move that Japan followed just three years later. And the US surgeon general in 2023 declared a loneliness crisis, a development that was extensively covered in the American media.[4] Yet, despite the attention surrounding the surgeon general's announcement, the only formal governmental position in the United States created in its wake was the appointment of the sex therapist Dr. Ruth Westheimer as New York State's honorary ambassador to loneliness, though even that job has remained unfilled since Dr. Ruth's death in 2024.

When it comes down to actual action and priorities, the reality of how we tackle healthy aging is still very focused on the physical: In much of the West—and really much of the world—healthy living is considered the responsibility of the individual and centers largely on physical care. It is about what I eat, how I exercise, how I sleep, and how I obtain my health care. Vast nutrition, fitness, and health care industries support that view of good health. I've seen it myself. In writing this book, I've had hundreds of conversations about healthy aging, and people invariably focus on diet, exercise, and health care. If I mention social health and its central role in healthy longevity, people tend to acknowledge its importance and then immediately shift the conversation back to the Mediterranean diet, the ten-thousand-step rule, or the impact of universal health care on public health. Ozempic by itself gets more airtime than social health.

While many people already acknowledge, or at least pay lip service to, the relevance of social connections to healthy longevity, few would elevate it to the same level of relevance as nutrition, fitness, and health care. Let's call it the 90/10 rule. In much of the West, 90 percent (though it's probably more like 99.9 percent) of our effort focuses on our bodily health: diet, nutrition, and exercise. You can fill Yucca Mountain with fad health books alone, as well as build several more waste repositories with the $37 billion that Americans spend each year on exercise equipment—a good chunk of which will be landfill anyway within a short period of time.

It is a big miss, because the evidence shows a critical, even paramount, link between social capital and healthy longevity. The first breakthrough in the area came in 1979 when two researchers—Lisa Berkman of Harvard and Leonard Syme of Berkeley—published the results of a nine-year study of almost seven thousand adults and found that loneliness increased mortality, independent of health condition, socioeconomic status, or behaviors like drinking or smoking.[5] Hundreds of studies since have confirmed the close connection between social connection and healthy aging—and the punishing impact of loneliness. And it's not just among specific populations, like White men from Boston. A 1988 study reported in the journal *Science*, for instance, tried to get at the universality of the measure by evaluating and synthesizing five studies conducted in different parts of the world: Evans County, Georgia; Alameda County in Northern California; Tecumseh Township in Michigan; Gothenburg in Sweden; and eastern Finland. Not surprisingly, there were enormous health and life expectancy differences between, for instance, a rural county in Georgia and a booming city in Sweden best known for its Volvos and its literary festival. But one thing held true across all the studies and whether the group was primarily White or heavily Black, or whether it was rich or poor, rural or urban: "People who were more socially connected had less risk of dying at any age."[6]

That finding has been replicated countless times throughout the intervening decades. In 2010, Julianne Holt-Lunstad, a professor at Brigham Young University, looked at 148 studies conducted in countries all over the world (including Canada, Denmark, Germany, China, Japan, and Israel, among others) and found that social connection had the same impact on health across all of them. Building on the prior works of Berkman and Syme, Holt-Lunstad quantified the association and found that social connection increased the likelihood of surviving in any given year by more than 50 percent.[7] Based on these findings, she concluded that social health, or lack thereof, is of greater health consequence than obesity and *equivalent to smoking fifteen cigarettes a day*. Other researchers have subsequently found that the effect of social health is equal to or greater than everything from physical inactivity to high blood pressure, cholesterol levels, air pollution, and clinical interventions such as the flu vaccine.[8]

Social connection and social fitness are particularly important to health in the second half of life, when we are most vulnerable to the loss of social networks and the rise of social isolation. During my research for this book, I traveled across Spain, reporting on its extraordinary success in longevity. It is already one of the longest-lived countries on Earth, and it is projected by some to have the longest life expectancy in the world by 2040. People in Spain, I found, are rather proud of their longevity. The idea of aging healthy to 100 is increasingly popular in Spain, reflected in the civic pride in the growing number of centenarians in the country. It's a good thing that the Spaniards love their centenarians because they have a whole lot of them: close to twenty thousand now, a number that is expected to rise to 373,000 within the next forty years.[9]

As I was crisscrossing Spain, researchers at the Universidad Politécnica de Madrid released a study of super-agers, a group defined as people with memory abilities comparable to those twenty to thirty years younger. Super-agers are a source of endless fascination to some researchers, but it's a hard group to study, largely because you need a place with lots and lots of old people in order to find a critical mass of them. Spain is a gold mine in that respect, and the Madrid researchers were able to recruit 119 centenarians, roughly half of whom fell in the category of super-agers. The other half had aged normally—though still well enough to hit the 100-year mark. The differences between the two groups? There was little difference in diet; the amount of sleep, alcohol intake, or tobacco use; fitness regimens; or even work backgrounds. Equivalent numbers in both groups ate a careful Mediterranean diet, while others subsisted on ultra-processed and fast foods. The only difference researchers were able to identify between the super-agers and their normally aging counterparts was that the super-agers had higher rates of social connection and lower rates of loneliness.

There are a number of reasons why we undervalue the importance of social connection to health and longevity: It's hard to measure—my Fitbit doesn't recognize it—and it's also hard to understand why it matters so much. It's easy to understand the impact of smoking once you've seen a lung X-ray, or to envision how a poor diet raises the risk of stopping your heart once you've learned how cholesterol and fats can clog up key coronary pathways, but there simply aren't such neat diagrams to sum up the multiple ways that social connection supports good health—and how loneliness undermines it. That's because social health is a precursor condition: In and of itself it is not a clinical condition, but it impacts a wide range of other conditions, from cardiovascular diseases to hypertension to diabetes and even infectious diseases.

Evolutionarily, humans are social creatures, biologically wired for social connection and common purpose. Throughout our history, the ability of humans to rely on one another—for food, shelter, and common protection—has been critical to survival and human flourishing. Our brains have adapted to expect and need proximity to others, because being outside the group was dangerous and a sign that we would have to perform the difficult tasks of survival all on our own. Our body responds to feelings of loneliness and chronic isolation by flooding our biological systems with stress signals.[10] This type of evolutionary response was built up over millions of years, and the relatively few years of our modern society have not dulled it.

Our bodies react to stress with increased inflammation. Stress and inflammation can go up and down with the vicissitudes of life, but chronic stress and inflammation, such as that caused by loneliness, can have a pervasive and negative effect on everything from cardiovascular disease to cancer, diabetes, depression, and Alzheimer's disease, as well as a variety of mental and cognitive health outcomes.[11] Research on the causal links between social health and mortality is still developing, but it is considered likely that inflammation is the common pathway that explains the many diverse health outcomes associated with isolation and loneliness.

There is also a correlative effect between social connection and health. At its most basic level, social connection gets people out of the house and moving, a basic signpost of healthy aging. But it's more than that: People with better social health markers are more likely to adopt better health behaviors, everything from reduced smoking and drinking to more exercise and better treatment adherence, including the taking of medicines and following health protocols. Social influence plays an important role in this—from a friend or relative urging better self-care to social cues about better behavior around everything from vaccinations to exercise. To be fair, social cues can have negative health impacts as well—witness all the social pressures that developed against taking the COVID-19 vaccine in some communities—but on balance they play a positive and often determinative role in healthy aging.

———

I live in Washington, DC, but I really began thinking about social health somewhere along O'Reilly Street, a dusty little thoroughfare that passes for the main drag in Presidio, Texas. Perhaps you're not familiar with Presidio. It's tiny, a little over three thousand people, and you're not likely to just blunder upon it. To get there from Washington, I had to fly to Houston, changing time zones from Eastern to Central time; then fly to El Paso, changing time zones again from Central to Mountain; and then drive back three hours, reverting again to Central time. You have to really want to go to Presidio to get there.

And I did. Not because I wanted to find out how an O'Reilly ended up in this almost entirely Latino town just across the border from Chihuahua, Mexico, but because Presidio was the first stop of a new season for the *Century Lives* podcast I host for the Stanford Center on Longevity. The season, which we had dubbed "Place Matters," was focused on outlier communities, places in the US that had better health results than the underlying data indicates they should. In the United States, there is an almost arithmetic correlation between county income and life expectancy. Raj Chetty, a social scientist based at Harvard, has done extensive research in the area and demonstrated that the richer the county, the higher the life expectancy and sadly the converse is also true: the poorer the county, the lower the life expectancy.[12] That's not all that surprising and is hardly unique to the United States, but what is astonishing is the level of dedication that almost every county in the US has to this formula. If you make a graph, as Chetty has done, with income on one axis and life expectancy on the other, and then draw a line up and to the right, virtually all of the 3,143 counties in the US cling to that line, as if the line is magnetic and the counties are made of metal. There are a handful of outliers, though remarkably few, and Presidio County is the outlier of all outliers. It's one of the poorest counties in Texas, among the bottom 5 percent in the entire country, but it still has the tenth-highest life expectancy of any county in the US. When it comes to longevity, there is no other place in the US like Presidio County.[13]

It's easy to cross off the things that don't explain good health in Presidio. It's not health care. There is little in the way of medical services in town, and the nearest American hospital is in Alpine, a bumpy seventy-mile drive away. It's not the diet, which was described to me as a traditional Mexican one, heavy on lard, fats, and cheeses, and that's certainly what I was offered at El Patio restaurant when we stopped in for dinner the first night in town. And it's not exercise: The principal of the high school is considered the local eccentric because he occasionally rides his bicycle through town. What does explain the high life expectancy in Presidio is social connection—and the intergenerational bonds that tie families and the community together. Many people live in multigenerational homes: parents, children, grandparents. And if they don't live in the same house, they live in family neighborhoods: brothers, sisters, aunts, uncles, cousins, grandparents all living on the same block, in and out of one another's houses all day, the doors unlocked, the kitchens open to anyone who drops in. It's a community evocative of decades long past, or of societies distant from the US, and it is the wellspring for the remarkable longevity in Presidio.

The story was the same wherever we turned up that season: places as dissimilar as Wayne County, Kentucky; Birmingham, Alabama; and Co-op City in the Bronx. The places were rural and urban, White and Black and Latino, poor and middle-income, and yet they all shared a common trait that residents were more socially engaged and more community-involved than in comparable areas—and were healthier because of it. Social science research is great—who can resist kicking back with a great longitudinal study—but it pales in comparison to seeing the impact of social connection in real life.

That's the good news. The bad news is that most of the other 3,139 counties are going in the wrong direction when it comes to social health, and you can see it in the life expectancy numbers in the US, and to a lesser extent in the UK. Average life expectancy in the US is only seventy-nine, a number that is lower than Japan, Singapore, and Spain by about six years, and largely indistinguishable from countries like Panama and Jordan, to mention just two nations that have far less resources and wealth than the United States. In a country as big and complicated as the US, gross statistics can mask considerable diversity of experience, but not for life expectancy. Women in the US trail their peers overseas, both in terms of life expectancy at birth and life expectancy at sixty, and the same is true for men. And it's not income disparities that explain the difference. Poor Americans lag behind poor people in other developed countries, and our middle class and wealthy also trail behind their respective financial peers—and the same is true if you have access to high-quality health care or if you don't.

But more important than just life expectancy are the measures of *healthy* life expectancy, and the US does even worse there, as the average American lives twelve and a half years in poor health, compared to a little over eleven in the UK, ten in Japan, nine and a half in Singapore, and under nine in China.[14] Because of this, a person raised in Singapore or Tokyo rather than, say, Chicago has the odds of a better part of a decade more of good health. It's really a stunning number, and if you are an American like me, it's a profound indictment of how we live our lives.

It wasn't always this way. Until the late 1970s and early 1980s, life expectancy in the United States was more or less equivalent to that of the other advanced economies of Western Europe and Asia. It wasn't the highest in the group typically, but it also wasn't the lowest, as it is now. But unobserved except by only a few, about forty-five years ago it began to diverge, with American health measures falling further and further behind those of peer nations. It wasn't a random development, as Bob Putnam, yet another one of those ubiquitous Harvard professors, described in his book *Bowling Alone*.[15] In the '70s and '80s, all the institutions that brought people together, creating social capital and connection, began to pull apart and decline. Religious activity began its long, slow descent, as did union membership. Participation in parent-teacher associations, which peaked at almost 50 percent in 1960, plunged to under 20 percent by 1980. Club meeting attendance fell by half, as did engagement in activities as diverse as attending a political rally or joining a sewing circle.

What replaced these group endeavors was a new tide of solitary activities. Putnam famously picked his book title from a story about how people were eschewing league participation in favor of bowling by themselves, but it was really technology that began the process of isolating us from one another. As early as 1950, people who had televisions watched them in huge quantity, about four hours per day, but the impact was muted overall, as only 9 percent of American households had televisions. But over the next three decades, television became more ubiquitous, and we began spending more time watching, pushing out congregational and participatory activities. By 1980, about 99 percent of households had televisions, and we watched an almost unfathomable amount—over seven hours per day. Today, we watch less television, though still almost three hours per day, but those saved hours (and then some) have been plowed right into the internet. Americans spend six hours and forty minutes per day on the internet, roughly forty-seven hours per week or seventeen years of an average person's adult life. It's a disconcerting number, though to be fair, it is not entirely unusual now: South Africans, Brazilians, and Filipinos spend over nine hours a day on the internet. But people in many (though not all) of the healthiest countries spend far less time online: Average use in Japan is under four hours per day, and Italy is under three.

———

While the US was heading in the wrong direction, other countries have been making tremendous strides—unparalleled in human history—in terms of collective health and life expectancy. In the summer of 1976, my parents bundled up our family—me, my older brother, Michael, and our fat little dog, Chevy—and moved us to South Korea, where my father had been newly posted to the US embassy. Coming from a leafy suburb of Washington, DC, the move was a bit of a shock to my middle school sensibilities, though I loved it. Seoul was noisy, chaotic, and confusing, but also splashed in color and brimming with energy. Korea was just emerging from a postwar malaise that had lasted two decades, and Seoul reverberated with possibilities. It seemed like everyone was selling something: pots and pans, knockoff Adidas runners, genuine Korean "antiques." Napolean might have disparaged the place as "a nation of shopkeepers," as he famously said of the British, but it would have been more accurate to call the Seoul of that time a city of "stall keepers," since most of the commercial action took place in open-air marketplaces scattered across the sprawling city. The place had a proto-capitalist feel to it, though if you squinted really hard you could see the outlines of the major manufacturing powerhouse that it would eventually become. Even in the 1970s, Korea already had a domestic automobile manufacturing sector, led by an obscure company called Hyundai that made rather unattractive and rickety small sedans. For us, Hyundais were an intriguing curiosity, though you would never buy one if you could afford, for instance, an Oldsmobile.

There was (and still is) much to admire in Korea. But it was still largely an isolated and economically underdeveloped society. There was little Western business presence, reflecting how far out of the global business flow it was at the time, and my brother was scandalized that there were no McDonald's in the country—a sure sign of social and economic backwardness. And that was reflected in broader social indicators like wealth, education, access to health care—and life expectancy. When we moved to Seoul, life expectancy in Korea was just sixty-three, a full nine years less than the United States at the time.

Little did I realize that our years in Seoul were the beginning of epochal changes, not just the coming flattening in health and life expectancy in the US that I just chronicled, but a surge in life expectancy in South Korea. Today, forty-eight years later, really a snap of the finger in human history, Koreans have added twenty-one years to life—and now can expect to live six years longer than Americans and four more than Brits. These numbers are unprecedented, shocking really, to anyone who studies human demography closely. But perhaps that doesn't sound all that impressive to you. Try to look at it this way: In less than half a century, the Koreans have added more years to life than they did in all of recorded human history before 1850, when the current boom in life expectancy began.

The story of life expectancy in Korea is truly extraordinary, but the fascinating thing is that it is not quite unique. Sixty years ago, life expectancy in Singapore was only sixty-six, about four years less than in the US and five years less than its former colonial overseers in the UK. In many ways, Singapore was an even less likely candidate for great strides in health and longevity than Korea. The city had prospered in the first decades of the twentieth century as the "Gibraltar of the East," a British fortress built to deter Japanese expansionism. That did not work out quite as the British planned, and the city swiftly fell to the Japanese in the early days of World War II. Tens of thousands of civilians and captured soldiers died under a brutal Japanese occupation, and the city's infrastructure was decimated. What emerged after World War II was a bleak, hollow, and mistrustful city, eager to see the backs of the British who had failed them so miserably, but deeply uncertain of its ability to survive on its own. Soon after the end of World War II, the British colonial government initiated a gradual transfer of power to local rule—a long, ugly process marked by ethnic tensions, economic jealousies, and disagreement about what to do with a territory that was more than a city but less than a country. Finally, in 1963, the issue was decided in favor of joining the newly created Malaysia, which combined Malaya, Singapore, North Borneo, and Sarawak into an independent federation. It went poorly. The new federation was riven with the same unresolved rivalries that characterized the end of the colonial period, and after just two years, the Malay central government took the unprecedented step of kicking Singapore out of the federation, thereby creating one of the smallest and most ill-prepared countries on Earth.

Accidental countries tend not to flourish, and very few observers thought the fledgling nation of Singapore would survive. Even Lee Kuan Yew, the country's leader at independence and for many decades afterward, declared the country at independence "a political, economic, and geographic absurdity."[16] Unemployment was rampant. Of its 1.9 million people, 1.3 million lived on the city's fringes mostly in squatter huts lacking modern sanitation, electricity, and water. It was not even a recipe for survival, let alone success. Yet over the last half century, Singapore has flourished: economically and demographically. The country has added eighteen years to life and is now not only one of the longest-lived countries in the world, but, in combination with Japan, it's the place where you would live if you wanted to have the longest *and* healthiest life.

Japan, Spain, and Italy have all followed similar, if not quite as dramatic, arcs, adding roughly fifteen years to life in each instance and being among the world's leaders in both life expectancy and healthy life expectancy. What knits these countries together is not just their extraordinary success in extending healthy life—there are, after all, other countries that have similar if not quite equal health results—but how they have done it. All these countries—sometimes intentionally, sometimes not—have put social health at the centerpiece of their public health strategies. They have done that through a cultural revolution in how to imagine the second half of life. All of these societies have rejected an outdated notion of the three-stage life: education to roughly twenty, work until sixty-five, and then retirement until death. Instead, these societies have arrived at a common place of a more fluid life course, one in which there is no magic cutoff between the years of health and productivity and the era of old age. The years past sixty-five, it is believed, should be part of productive adulthood and not just a long, steepening decline into death. Long-life health means shifting the concept of aging and realizing that traditionally "old" people can now stay productive as long as they are afforded the opportunities to stay engaged, learn, and remain vital parts of their community. It is, to borrow a phrase from the Stanford Center on Longevity, a new map of life, a new set of rules for how we conduct our supersized lives.[17]

Reconceiving the life course is critical but not sufficient. Cultural and mindset changes are the necessary first step, but building a social health infrastructure is also important in keeping older adults connected and flourishing. Want to improve your nutrition? Or your cardiovascular fitness? There are things that society can provide to make that easier, but essentially, you can do it on your own. Social health is different. It is fundamentally a team sport and requires social norms and social infrastructure that maximize the opportunities for social health, and ultimately healthy longevity.

Over the first half of 2024, I traveled to five of the most successful aging countries in the world—Japan, Korea, Spain, Italy, and Singapore—to see how these societies are working to keep older people (and really the entire population) active, engaged, connected, and purposeful—and healthy as a result. I chose these five countries because they are the healthiest and longest-lived in the world (though a few other countries like Switzerland could sneak onto that list if that was the only criteria) and because they are geographically, socially, and economically diverse—and as a group don't rank at the top of indicators such as GDP, exercise, and obesity that are often said to predict health and life expectancy. In these countries, I encountered very different cultural and economic differences, but I discovered key commonalities around changing norms of work, lifelong learning, intergenerational relationships, and volunteerism, all nested in a growing embrace of a more active, productive, and engaged second half of life.

After my family returned home from Korea in 1979, I'd sometimes watch the *Today* show with my mother, who often had it on in the background as she went about her morning routine. We had a small amount of civic pride in the fact that Willard Scott, our local weatherman, had ascended to the national stage. Scott was big, round, and jovial, and his charm lay less in his weather forecasting abilities and more in his congenial personality and his relationship with the people around him. Beginning in 1983, in addition to reporting the weather, he began offering on-air birthday wishes to anyone who was hitting the century mark that day. He could devote valuable airtime because turning 100 was an outlier event, reserved for the special few who somehow surpassed normal demographic limits. But that was then. During my travels I was struck by the views across these healthy countries that the 100-year life is moving from an extraordinary event worthy of national notice to an ordinary benchmark of how long life should be. And that's reflected in the numbers. According to the United Nations, there were only twenty-three thousand centenarians in the world in 1950, a number which had ballooned to 110,000 by 1990 and 593,000 by 2022. But that's just the beginning, as the UN predicts that there will be 3.7 million centenarians worldwide by 2050, 440,000 of them in Japan alone.[18] That's a 160-fold increase in just a century, and it means that there will be more centenarians in Japan alone than there were in the entire world a few years ago.

Not everyone in even the healthiest places—far from it—will soon live to 100 in good health. But it is the case that such an idea is not so fanciful as it once seemed—the median life expectancy for women in Japan is already ninety, and studies have suggested that half the children born today will live to 100 if life expectancy increases continue on their current trajectory.[19] The idea of a century-long life is an increasingly common reference point for long life, and there exists a shared notion across all the successful aging countries I visited that those ten decades of life can be healthy and productive ones. Healthy to 100 is no longer the stuff of fables but increasingly a reasonable aspirational goal for individuals and communities alike.

Critical to this idea is the convergence between life expectancy and healthy life expectancy. All times of life come with specific challenges, and later life is no different, bringing with it a set of physical and cognitive risks unique to that stage. No advances in medical or social sciences will eliminate those frailties anytime soon, but healthy to 100 means reducing the odds of long periods of physical decline and maximizing the opportunity for healthy living to, or very close to, the end. Increasingly, the healthiest countries in the world are making progress toward that goal not as a function of stepped-up investments in health care but by creating a social infrastructure that supports community, connection, and purpose throughout our longer lives.

In the coming pages, we will explore the research that connects good health with social capital and social connections: with having a wide network of friends, coworkers, and casual acquaintances; with intergenerational relationships; with volunteering and having a sense of purpose and mission; with caregiving and close family bonds. And we will explore what the healthiest nations in the world are doing to maximize that opportunity for social health and what you can take away as lessons for yourself, your family, and your community.

When it comes to healthy aging, it always seems that other countries know things we don't know here in the US. There is undoubtedly some truth to that, as cultural value systems matter enormously, but it is equally the case that necessity is the mother of invention. The five countries that I am profiling here not only have very high life expectancy rates but also some of the lowest birth rates in the world. Korea has the lowest birth rate, now significantly under one child per woman (about .7) over the course of her adult life.[20] That's less than half of the birth rate in the US and the UK and very far from the 2.1 children per woman rate needed to keep the population steady. The combination of rising life expectancy and collapsing birth rate means that these societies are getting older on a scale unprecedented in human history; already, 30 percent of Japan's population is over the age of sixty-five, and 10 percent is over the age of eighty—and Italy is not far behind. As recently as 2015, the ratio in Japan between people in the core working ages of fifteen to sixty-four to those aged sixty-five and older was 2.2. By 2040, that number will plunge to 1.5. All of this means that these societies will not be able to flourish if practices around aging, work, and lifelong health are not dramatically changed. It is little wonder that these countries have furiously innovated to keep their graying populations healthy, productive, and engaged, because it is likely not just a matter of population health but of societal survival. The economic and demographic imperatives in the US may be different, or at least we may lag behind a bit on those risks, but we still have a unique opportunity to learn the critical lessons on how to maximize collective and personal health.

———

The idea of living healthy to 100 (or beyond) is not a new one. Rather, it reflects a universal longing that has echoes in literature and legend and reflects our aspirations for balancing out the definitiveness and completeness of death. It's why the idea of a Fountain of Youth has found such purchase both over time and geography.

Most Americans and Europeans associate the concept of the Fountain of Youth with the Spaniard Juan Ponce de León and his explorations of Florida. Ponce de León was a Spanish nobleman, a confederate of Christopher Columbus and a rival to Columbus's son, Diego Colón. He was an influential figure in the New World but was bested by Colón in a long-drawn-out court battle over the right to govern Puerto Rico. Licking his wounds, Ponce de León turned to King Ferdinand and sought—and received—royal authority to lay claims to rumored lands to the north of Puerto Rico, lands that Ponce de León dubbed La Florida during his first journey of discovery. In 1513, he set out from Puerto Rico with three ships, the *Santiago*, the *San Cristobal*, and the *Santa Maria de la Consolación*, and within weeks he had spied Florida. On April 3, Ponce de León came ashore in a spot that is generally thought to be near St. Augustine, grandly claiming the lands in the name of the Spanish monarchy but mostly in the hopes that he would be able to personally exploit the natural resources of the territory.

Exploiting natural resources is an expensive proposition, though, and it took Ponce de León many years to raise sufficient funds for the venture. It wasn't until 1521 that he was able to return along with two hundred settlers and fifty horses plus homesteading and farming equipment, planning to create a longer-term presence in Florida. Unfortunately for Ponce de León, the Calusa Indians who controlled that area of Southwestern Florida had other ideas. They fiercely resisted the settlers, and Ponce de León was struck by a poison-tipped arrow, forcing a retreat to Havana, where he died of his wounds.

There are a number of contemporaneous accounts of Ponce de León's two trips to Florida, both from his own hand and those around him, and they differ in many details but are consistent in one critical way: None of them mention in any way the search for or the discovery of a Fountain of Youth. It wasn't until 1535 that the Spanish historian Oviedo wrote that Ponce de León was seeking to regain his youthfulness with the waters of Bimini, an island described in Caribbean lore as a place of great wealth and longevity.

Later historians picked up Oviedo's account, and over the centuries Ponce de León has become synonymous with the concept of the Fountain of Youth and the intrinsic human desire to live not only for an extraordinarily long time, but also to live those years in good health.

The myth of Ponce de León and the Fountain of Youth has been burnished over the years by a motley collection of characters, none more delightful than Luella Day McConnell. McConnell, or "Diamond Lil" as she came to be known, was an adventurer and a wild inventor of fables—she would almost certainly be a successful social media influencer if she were alive today. Born in the second half of the nineteenth century, McConnell claimed to be a medical doctor who had sought her fortune in the Yukon gold rush. In 1904 she resettled to St. Augustine, and in 1909, conveniently coincident with an uptick in popular interest in the Ponce de León story, she announced that she had discovered a natural spring, happily located in her front yard, that corresponded to his Fountain of Youth.[21] Diamond Lil reported at the time that a tree next to her well had fallen down, exposing a stone arrangement in the shape of a cross, fifteen feet long by thirteen feet across, marking the year that Ponce de León had come ashore. Next to the cross, according to McConnell, was a silver urn embossed with an image of Columbus and containing a parchment said to be written by a member of Ponce de León's crew. The urn disappeared and the parchment became unreadable, but that did not stop McConnell's spring from becoming the most popular attraction in St. Augustine. The Fountain of Youth made Diamond Lil a prominent fixture in St. Augustine and a source of much local news and gossip. But unfortunately for her, the Fountain of Youth had as little providential impact on her as it did on Ponce de León, as she died in a one-car accident in 1927.

A century on, McConnell's story seems comical and ludicrous, but if there is one thing we know about people, it is that they will believe what they want—and for centuries, people have wanted to believe in magical sources that promise eternal or at least very long life. Well before Ponce de León, tales of magical springs of longevity captivated Europeans. In the fifth century BCE, Herodotus, the Greek historian and geographer, wrote of the Macrobians, who were believed to have lived in modern-day Africa and were renowned for their youthfulness. He ascribed their longevity to a mysterious pool of water that he speculated was the source of their great power.[22]

It's not just a European thing. The first emperor of unified China, Qin Shi Huang, was obsessed with the search for immortality, dispatching his emissaries far and wide in search of an elixir of life. The emperor made it clear to all that he would not brook failure in this quest. Hearing rumors that the alchemists who were providing potions for him may not have been as fully confident in their success as they claimed to be, he rounded up 460 alchemists, scientists, and scholars and had them all buried alive, making rather clear to the world that the search for immortality was more of a me thing than an us thing. Facing certain execution if they returned with empty hands, many of the emperor's agents quite sensibly disappeared and were never heard from again. Ironically, I would even say fittingly, modern researchers believe that Qin Shi Huang died from mercury poisoning, from pills that were proffered as miracle cures for an illness.[23]

Stories of healing waters—it's almost always water for some reason—can be found in the cultural archives of such geographically diverse societies as the Canary Islands, Japan, Polynesia, England, and Greece, and some tales have even ricocheted across nations and continents.[24] In the twelfth century, the exploits of a Christian king named Prester John swept across Europe, first enthralling the court of Manuel I Komnenos, the Byzantine emperor; then Pope Alexander III in Rome; and eventually Frederick Barbarossa, the Holy Roman emperor in Germany. Prester John's kingdom, it was said, was home to an extraordinary Fountain of Youth, which had permitted him to live in good health for more than five hundred years. In some of the retellings, it was also reported that all the people of Prester John's peaceable lands could drink from this life-giving fountain and live for 120 years, and sometimes much longer.

The idea that life could extend to 120 and beyond was both tantalizing and a little absurd at the time. Thomas Hobbes's famous account of civil life in *Leviathan* as "nasty, brutish, and short" was a particularly apt description of life in the Middle Ages. The average person in Europe during that period could expect to live only a little more than thirty years. Even the kings and queens of England and Scotland averaged only about forty-eight years, not particularly surprising given frequent wars, the absence of sanitation, and a medical community that believed disease needed to be drained from the body through bleeding, cupping, and leeching. The idea that both royalty and ordinary people could live to 120 or even close to that was both a beguiling and fantastical notion.

It's easy to dismiss the search for the Fountain of Youth as the product of a more credulous and less scientific time, but in a way, we are still looking for modern versions of the Fountain of Youth, now cloaked as medical and biological moon shots. Ever since 1993 when Cynthia Kenyon, a molecular biologist and biogerontologist

at the University of California San Francisco, made the discovery
that a single gene mutation could double the lifespan of ordinary
roundworms, a new generation of tech millionaires and billion-
aires, almost always men, have latched with great zeal onto the idea
that "aging is a disease, and that disease is treatable." Bold-face tech
titans such as Bezos, Thiel, Altman, and Zuckerberg have invested
heavily in start-ups such as Altos Labs that seek to perfect cellular
reprogramming as part of a leap forward strategy on human longevity. They believe that technology can solve the problem of death,
just as they once believed that it would solve poverty, hunger, and
the ills of government. Whether it is changes to diet, the use of supplements, or breakthroughs in T cells or gene therapies, the goal is
age reversal and extra-long life, if not quite an immortal one.

Perhaps they will reach immortality, but people who have
sought immortality or the nearest available option are more likely to
be cautionary tales than record-breakers. Supercentenarians (those
who live past 110) are rarely people impassioned about living super
long lives. They are more typically average people with strong social
connections, good support systems, and lives of purpose and meaning. I've interviewed supercentenarians and centenarians from time
to time, and they share a zest for life rather than the fear of death
that seems to animate the billionaire class.

I am not the first person to seek lessons on healthy aging from other
countries. I was frequently asked during my research whether I was
writing another Blue Zones book. For those not familiar with the
Blue Zones concept (a dwindling number after Netflix aired a doc-
umentary series about it in 2023), it is the name given to a small

number of mostly isolated and rural places around the world where good diets, low-stress environments, and other healthy habits are claimed to lead to startling long life. There are open questions about the reliability of the life expectancy data in these places, but even if recordkeeping in Sardinia and the Nicoya Peninsula in Costa Rica may not be all that you would want, the basic lessons are still pretty compelling.[25] Dan Buettner, the author who popularized the Blue Zone concept, attributed their success to the slow pace of life, a close connection with nature, and the abundance of fresh, local foods such as coconuts, squash, and beans. The lessons from these Blue Zones have positively impacted how we think about longevity, especially in the areas of food and diet—but in practice they have proven difficult to transfer to many of our busy, complicated, modern lives.

And that's the difference between the Blue Zones and this book. This book in some ways is intended to be the antithesis of the Blue Zones, because virtually everyone reading this book lives in a place completely *unlike* a traditional Blue Zone, and that is not likely to change. Most of us don't eat nut- and bean-based diets, our work lives are often high-stress, and I don't recall any cooling trade winds wafting across center-city Washington, DC. It would be lovely if we all did live in a Blue Zone, but we can't. And if we all tried to move to a Blue Zone, it would create not good things for us but bad things for traditional practices in the Blue Zones. In fact, that's exactly what is happening in Okinawa and Nicoya as modernity encroaches on traditional practices in what have typically been distant and isolated communities. As the Nicoya Peninsula, for instance, has become more closely connected with the rest of Costa Rica, it is not Costa Rica that has been influenced by Nicoya, but Nicoya that has been

changed by some of the unhealthier habits of modern, urban societies, to the possible detriment of health there.

The impressive part about industrialized, heavily urbanized,
and densely populated societies like Japan and Korea is not that
they have created perfect Blue Zone conditions for healthy aging,
but that they have succeeded despite suboptimal aging conditions. Everyone I interviewed for this book lives complicated lives
reflective of modern times and yet flourishes even in the context
of stressful and hectic urban life. Take Singapore, for instance. It's
a country renowned for its hot, crowded conditions, competitive
work environments, and—despite an incredibly diverse and exciting food scene—a national obsession with fast food. Singapore has
one of the highest concentrations of McDonald's in the world. Head
down any street and you might bump into a Shake Shack, a Pizza-
boy, a Fatburger, or, best yet, a Devil Chicken, where you can order
a Crispy Chicken Skin, for those who want to have all the fat and
grease of fried chicken without the bother of the meat.

Spain, unlike Singapore, is known for its more balanced
approach to life, but it's all relative, and Spain still bears the marks
of modern life. Obesity rates are high, income is well below the
European Union average, and smoking rates are among the highest
in Europe, almost 50 percent higher than in the US (though still
lower than Japan and South Korea). And none of these countries
are particularly good at exercise. In a World Economic Forum
study of exercise rates in twenty-nine advanced countries, Japan
ranked twenty-eighth, Italy was twenty-seventh, South Korea was
in the bottom quartile, and Spain was in the bottom half (Singapore was not rated). Yet it is these countries—not the UK, the US,
Canada, and Australia, all of whom were rated in the top half of

fitness—who are setting the standard for healthy aging. None of that is an endorsement of forsaking your morning run in favor of queuing up first thing at Mister Donut, as everyone in Singapore seems to do, but if these societies can foster healthy longevity even amid less-than-pristine conditions, surely there will be lessons that we can apply to our own lives.

———

Over the coming chapters, I'm going to lay out the lessons from my travels, and how we can improve our social health both individually and collectively. Each chapter will dive into one key pillar of social connection and try to distill the learnings that might help you age more healthfully. At times, I thought some of the things I was learning were almost painfully obvious, but I was frequently reminded that what might seem certain in Fukuoka, Japan, was not so clear back at home.

During a break in the travels for this book, my wife and I attended the wedding of Sarah and Jay, the daughter and (now) son-in-law of longtime friends. After the wedding ceremony, we all retired to an enormous tent for the reception and dinner. Beth and I wandered about, catching up with a few old friends and briefly hugging the parents of the bride before they scuttled off to attend to one wedding issue or another. I eventually made it to the little table containing seating assignments, plucked our card, and ushered Beth over to Table 23.

Dinner was served and the toasts began, following a familiar script. David, the younger brother of the bride, recalled how desperate he was as a child for the attention of his big sister: "I was so eager to hang out with her that I didn't even complain when she painted my toy cars with pink fingernail polish." It was funny, warm, and heartfelt, and the subsequent speeches followed in kind. Fond stories of childhood, light jabs at the idiosyncrasies of the bride and groom—"Sarah is always hot. Jay is always cold."—and then an honor roll of the great things that lie ahead for the next twenty years: honeymoon, a first home, kids, jobs, promotions, more promotions, hobbies, community, travel, and shared moments. It's a vision of a busy and purposeful life together, one that will unspool over the coming decades.

But at Table 23, tucked away in the back of the tent, the vibe was rather different. This was the outer ring of the wedding, the last of the twenty-three tables, physically a step down from the main floor as to acknowledge our separateness. And as it turns out, it was an apt arrangement since Table 23 was assigned to the friends of the bride's parents. We were "the olds" in a room where the centripetal force was centered on people at least a generation younger than us. And our conversation reflected the sense of separation. Instead of happy talk about the adventures and opportunities in store for us, the table conversation gravitated toward retirement and a goal of gearing down. It was an unusual conversation for a Washington crowd: The celebrities at our table weren't the people with the important government jobs; instead, they were the four people who had retired in the last year, a statistically reasonable distribution at a table in which the average age was roughly sixty years old.

We all eagerly quizzed the newly retired on what it was like, as if they were adventurers who had just taken a marvelous trip. When did you retire? What do you do? Is it amazing? Questions flew at the table heroes, with the unstated expectation that we were all supposed to be jealous of these newfound freedoms, just as at another table others might have been envious of a hike on the Inca Trail. Our newly retired friends were happy to share their stories. Andrea boasted of "reading books during daylight and not feeling guilty about it." Josie told us about volunteering for the board of her local theater company (though it was teetering on the verge of bankruptcy in these post-pandemic days and might not be around for her second term), and the mother of the bride's law school roommate's husband bragged about learning to cook those dishes he never had time for before.

We all oohed and aahed, it would have been churlish not to, but in truth it was all thin, maybe even pitifully thin, stuff. It was impossible not to notice the difference between the extensive plans of Sarah and Jay, decades stuffed with goals and ideas and purpose, and the virtually nonexistent agenda for what could be decades of retirement. It's a common story—a life full of goals, plans, accomplishments, and responsibilities, and then it all stops. Our social networks, often built around work or schooling, fade away and for too many people, the hours of the day become owned by television, Instagram, and the emptiness of social isolation. I'm not saying that will happen to my chums at Table 23. Maybe Andrea will flourish reading one great book after another, but it is too common of a story to discount.

The irony of Table 23 is hard to avoid. Most everyone at the table, if I read the room correctly, were high achievers, people who excelled at school and in work: the type of people who planned careers and lives with meticulous care. They are Sarah and Jay thirty years on. But some deep cultural biases have told them that the next twenty years are less worthwhile than the twenty before those and the twenty before that. In truth, if you hit sixty in good health, as all my tablemates appeared to have done, your odds of another healthy twenty or more years are pretty good. Jay and Sarah are full of plans and ideas for their next twenty, but something has stopped the people of Table 23 from treating their next twenty with the same seriousness of purpose and care. As I picked at my tuna and faked a few huzzahs for retirement, my mind was silently screaming, "What are you going to do with all that time on your hands?"

The problem facing Table 23 is that there is no blueprint, no plan, no social infrastructure for connection as we age. Most everyone at the table is reaching some great tipping point in their life. Kids are leaving home, employers are signaling it's time to get out, connections built over a lifetime are beginning to stretch and fade. It is precisely the moment for people to try to step forward in their community, to engage more, but society is telling them instead that it is time to fall back. Our crisis of social isolation and loneliness is certainly not a product of one moment in the great continuum of life, but if it was, this would be it.

It's not that way everywhere, as I discovered on my travels. The most successful aging countries in the world view these years differently—as years of productivity, value, and purpose. This is a book about how these forward-looking countries are building a new vision of that second half of life and have created a social infrastructure to support connections that will help older adults make the next twenty years as valuable and meaningful as the last. This is a story of countries that have hit the age tunnel before us and are coming out the other end with a very different view of how we can be healthy to 100.

While one strand of the coming chapters will focus on what society must do to support social health, you don't have to wait for society to come around. At the end of each chapter, I'm going to offer actionable steps to improve social health. I will offer these ideas with some hesitation, because of course the best plans will differ based upon individual circumstances. You might be twenty or eighty, working or retired, an American or a Brit or Indian. There are universal principles, of course, but I'm not going to pretend that I have the "one size fits all" plan here for everyone.

But I do have a way of targeting my advice. Threaded throughout the book will be recommendations developed specifically for the people of Table 23. My tablemates were all in their fifties and sixties, some working, some retired, but all nearing an inflection point where they will be making choices, or defaulting into choices, about how they want to spend the next twenty years—and whether it will be a next act or something far more passive than that. Much of the advice will, I believe, have value far beyond the specific demographics of Table 23, but you, dear reader of indeterminate age, geography, and status, can evaluate the advice for your own individual circumstance. It's a journey, but if we take that journey together, perhaps next time when I am at Table 23, the people there will be as full of plans, ideas, and as many hopes for the future as Sarah and Jay.

Chapter 1

Hurry, Hurry

VEN AT 9:00 p.m. on a Thursday night, after a two-hour
lecture, the auditorium buzzes with energy. Questions
fly from the audience about healthy life expectancy, the
retirement age, lifelong learning, and the challenges of an aging
society, until finally the dean mercifully signals that the event has
reached its end. I'd like to think it is my lecture that has everyone
all ginned up—who isn't turned on by a talk on the American life
expectancy disadvantage—but it's a shade more likely the excitement stems from the fact that this is the first ever school-wide event
for the brand-new School of Future Life at Kyungnam University in
Changwon, Korea.[1]

Giving a talk, especially a jumbo-sized one like this, typically
takes my full attention, but the translation process here affords
me welcome breaks in the action. The questions from the audience come in Korean and are translated into English. I respond
in English, and then let my eyes wander over the audience as my
answers are converted back to Korean. I can see right away that it's

not your typical university audience, maybe 100 people, with ages ranging from twenty-five to about eighty, the majority landing in their fifties, sixties, and early seventies.

The audience is brimming with energy, but after two hours of talking, I'm not. I had taken the KTX, the Korean version of the bullet train, from Seoul early that morning down to Changwon, a city of about one million people near the bottom tip of the Korean Peninsula. I had been met at the train station by Kyung Hi Kim, an American-trained academic, a professor of education at Kyung-nam, and the new head of the School of Future Life. I thought that I might get a little downtime before my talk, or at least time to check into my hotel, but Kyung Hi had other ideas. She whisked me off to a late lunch, squired me around on a rapid tour of the town and the university, then ushered me to a meeting with the town's deputy mayor, and from there, took me directly to an improbably early dinner with student leaders. You might think that such a tight schedule is a bit insensitive to the weary traveler, but it all makes a certain logic in a country whose motto of "pali-pali" can be roughly translated as "hurry hurry."

You can apply that same motto to the School of Future Life, as it is a symbol of the rapid shift in Korea from an educational effort focused, as it is in most of the world, on grades K–12 (plus college) to a lifelong model where people are encouraged to learn throughout their lives. It is a shift from a notion that education is meant to prepare you for life to an idea that education is a critical part of living: an ingredient of personal development, health, social inclusion, and active citizenship.

The idea of lifelong learning, and especially adult education, is not new or unique to Korea. The phrase can be traced back at least to the nineteenth century, and in early formulations, it was most often associated with these concepts of citizenship and personal development. Winston Churchill extolled the virtues of adult learning by pledging his government's support for anyone who has a "thirst in later life to learn about the humanities, the history of their country, the philosophies of the human race, and the arts and letters which sustain and are borne forward by the ever-conquering English language."

But in more recent decades, the idea of adult learning has both fortunately lost a bit of that manifest destiny flavoring and slightly less fortunately become closely associated with worker training, and the need to "upskill" workers in an era of rapid technology change. The focus on worker training in recent years has led to rapid increases in skills certification (there are now more than one million certification programs in the US alone)[2] and a parallel diminishment of the idea of learning as key to personal development and social cohesion. Witness Alan Johnson, the labour secretary of state for education and skills in the government of Tony Blair: "We need plumbers, less Pilates; to subsidize precision engineering not oversubsidized flower arranging, except of course where flower arranging is necessary for a vocational purpose! . . . Tai chi may be hugely valuable to people studying it, but it's of little value to the economy."[3] Few have put it quite so baldly as Johnson, but his view fairly captures the ascendency of skills training at the expense of learning for learning's sake.

That is not the view in Korea. Learning is perceived not just as a tool of production, but as a critical element in a well-rounded life of meaning, purpose, and personal enrichment. A right to lifelong learning was added to the Korean constitution in 1980, a rather

startling development for someone from a country where prohi-
bitions on quartering troops are in the constitution but rights to
education and housing, for instance, are not.[4] The right to lifelong
learning in Korea stems from a social indebtedness to a postwar
generation that helped rebuild Korea but missed out on the educational benefits of a modern economic power.

But the investments in lifelong learning also reflect a need to keep
older generations active, engaged, healthy, and productive. Korea
has a shockingly low birth rate. At about 0.7 births per woman, it's
the lowest in the world and not by a small amount—some 30 percent
lower than even other countries with low birth rates like Japan and
China and less than half of the US, the UK, and Germany. Massive
investments in childcare and subsidized housing (Seoul is now even
offering to pay men to reverse vasectomies)[5] have not altered the
downward plunge in birth rates. The scarcity of children has knocked
Korea off its demographic axis with occasional head-snapping consequences: Pet strollers outsold baby strollers in 2023, for instance.[6]
In a country increasingly composed of people over the age of fifty,
keeping that population productive and healthy is a critical task, and
lifelong learning is an important tool in the effort.

The Ministry of Education was handed the lifelong learning
portfolio in the late 1990s, and it has taken on the task with considerable zeal. Over the last quarter century, Korea has built up an
incredibly dense network of adult learning centers, making learning easily accessible to seniors and younger adults alike. Suwon, a
community of about 1.2 million, operates more than six hundred
learning centers spread across the city with the goal of ensuring that
no citizen needs to walk more than five or ten minutes to reach a
classroom.[7]

In 2023, the Ministry of Education declared that Korean universities should also be playing a larger role in adult education. To jump-start that effort, the ministry created a grant program for universities around the country to develop lifelong learning programs. There were many reasons for the central government to support this effort, not the least of which was to help shore up the business model of Korean universities at a time when declining birth rates were reducing the pool of young college applicants. But the primary driving force, reflective of broader Korean investments in learning, was to create new education outlets for older adults, many of whom had missed out on the possibility of a college education in the first place.

Kyungnam University was one of the first applicants to the program, and it moved with astonishing speed once it was awarded its first grant in the summer of 2023. In roughly eight months, the team at the new School of Future Life developed a curriculum, established six different degree tracks within the program, hired faculty, and recruited and enrolled an intergenerational cohort of 120 students. It is a dizzying effort that would be impossible in virtually all academic settings around the world but perhaps seems routine within the context of Korean work culture and pali-pali.

All of this gives the School of Future Life the feel of a gold rush town, as if the inhabitants just arrived and the buildings were erected overnight. Over dinner, I meet the two newly elected leaders of the student body. Kim whispers to me that it is her first meeting with them too—and it's not clear to me whether the student leaders have even met each other. That doesn't mean there aren't important preexisting relationships within the student body. After the talk, two students approach me (Kim did not know their names yet either), a mother and daughter who had both enrolled at Kyungnam and were making plans to get their PhDs in education together after they had completed their initial degrees. It's a reflection of the wide-ranging, intergenerational, and social aspirations of the School of Future Life, supporting both students (like the daughter) who are at the front end of their careers and students (like the mother) who are charting second careers or are primarily interested in learning for its social, intellectual, and health benefits.

For the oldest group of learners, the school offers an "active seniors" learning track, which includes courses focused on exercise, health, financial planning, and personal beauty. The course catalogue reads a little wonky to me, but Kim assures me that the goal is not to necessarily get everything perfect from the jump but to test what works, what doesn't, and make rapid adjustments as needed. It might be called iterative design here in the US, but in Korea it's just another element of hurry, hurry.

I am sufficiently steeped in the bureaucratic processes of academia and government in the US to be dazzled at the speed of implementation. It's impressive, for sure, but the speed is not what makes the School of Future Life so meaningful. The School of Future Life is just a new chapter for Korea in an ongoing effort to rethink learning as something that should be done routinely throughout the whole life—and not just in the first part. And that purpose, social engagement, and good health will flourish as a result.

———

It is not surprising, at least from one perspective, that the School of Future Life was able to fill its seats so quickly, especially with older learners. We have gradually grasped as a species that learning is important to cognitive health and can help ward off the scourges of late life, like Alzheimer's and dementia. Older Americans, for instance, regularly tell pollsters that they both like to learn and correctly connect it with brain health. And 68 percent of them think that life becomes stagnant without continuous learning.[8] Because of this, all sorts of activities are held up as opportunities to increase cognitive health: Wordle, crossword puzzles, sudoku, and virtually any type of online course.

And it's largely true. The human brain is a marvelous feat of evolutionary engineering—an infinitely complex instrument composed of some eighty-six *billion* neurons—but it's also surprisingly human. Isolate it, starve it of stimulation, bore it, and the brain will atrophy, taking you along with it. Nurture it, stimulate it, and give it a reason to go on, and the odds are far better that you will have a healthy, longer life.

That may now seem intuitive, but it is only in recent decades that scientists have begun to understand the powerful role that mental engagement plays in human health. In the late 1980s, researchers, mostly in the United States, began uncovering puzzling cases of individuals with no apparent symptoms of dementia who were nonetheless found at autopsy to have brain changes consistent with advanced Alzheimer's. It caused a sensation within the neurology community, and a number of working theories quickly emerged, were evaluated, and were ultimately discarded. Eventually, the medical community settled on a concept called "cognitive reserve."[9]

Think of cognitive reserve as the brain's ability to improvise and find alternative ways of getting a job done. Just like a car enables you to engage another gear and suddenly accelerate to avoid danger, the brain can change the way it operates and make added resources available to cope with challenges—especially the type of

challenges that come along in later life. Cognitive reserve is sometimes described as the brain's fifth gear, but, if we want to stick to the
automotive analogy, I prefer to think of it as a second gas tank that
will provide your brain with fuel for longer than you expect. It's the
Hanukkah of neurobiology.

Over the last forty years, scientists have found links between
cognitive reserve and the ability to stave off Parkinson's disease,
multiple sclerosis, and even strokes. A deeper cognitive reserve
can also help people function better for longer even when they are
exposed to unexpected life events, such as stress, surgery, or tox-
ins in the environment. How do you increase cognitive reserve and
brain plasticity? Exercise the brain. High levels of social interaction
help, as do educational activities such as learning a new language or
joining a book club.

The single most important study of cognitive reserve is the Nun
Study of Aging and Alzheimer's Disease, popularly short-handed as
the Nun Study.[10] In the mid-1980s, a graduate student at the University of Minnesota, a former nun herself, told one of her professors
about a group of aging nuns at the School Sisters of Notre Dame.
The information intrigued her professor, David Snowdon, then an
assistant professor of epidemiology, because he thought that they
might be uniquely interesting subjects for a planned study on the
factors that influence rates of Alzheimer's and dementia. Fundamentally, he was trying to find out which activities, jobs, or even
attitudes would impact cognitive abilities, and which wouldn't.

The School Sisters of Notre Dame offered a promising setup.
One of the biggest hurdles in longevity research is that people live
very different lives and are exposed to a wide variety of influences
that affect health and life expectancy; it's very difficult to isolate the

impact of any one variable. The challenge for researchers in this field is to identify and recruit a test population that lives in such a way as to reduce the number of variables. Snowdon had first considered working with prisoners and found much to recommend them: They dress alike, eat the same foods, and generally have the same sleep habits and exercise opportunities. But the idea proved unworkable because prisoners tend to have very short lives, and they sometimes get out of prison, undermining the consistency that is needed in longitudinal studies.

Snowdon quickly realized that the nuns offered an even better opportunity. They live in the same type of housing, eat the same foods, have the same limited access to drugs and alcohol, have identical marital and economic status, and even move in the very same social circles. And even better, since Snowdon was interested in studying people over the age of seventy-five, nuns have atypically high life expectancies, and most stay with their order and in their convents all the way to death. And to the extent that their lives varied—some of the nuns were teachers, some did more blue-collar work in the convent—they varied in a way that was relevant to the study. You really couldn't invent a better test group if you wanted to.

But there was a catch. Snowdon had some strict requirements for inclusion in the study. Participants had to give Snowdon permission to comb through their autobiographies that they had written when they entered the order, often a half century before; submit to regular and fairly rigorous physical and cognitive exams; and, most intrusively, allow Snowdon and his team to cut open and study their brains upon death. I don't know what it takes to convince a large number of elderly, cloistered nuns that they should authorize a total stranger to invade their private thoughts and cut their brains open.

I don't even know how you broach such a conversation, but Snowdon must have had extraordinary powers of persuasion as he eventually coaxed 678 nuns into joining the study.

For the last forty years, Snowdon and successive directors of the Nun Study have painstakingly studied this group of nuns: reading their journals, subjecting them to a battery of physical and mental tests, and conducting autopsies on the participants, at least the ones with the good manners to die during the study period. The findings from the Nun Study, spooled out over many years, reveal in layered ways the critical role of learning to cognitive and physical health—and the cumulative effect across the life course. Nuns who had greater education, who wrote personal statements and essays with greater complexity and word density, were all less likely to show evidence of Alzheimer's, dementia, or other significant cognitive impairments. And the differences were not small. About 80 percent of the nuns whose writings were deemed to be lacking in linguistic density ultimately developed Alzheimer's or other dementia in old age, compared to a mere 10 percent diagnosis rate among those who evidenced more sophisticated and complex writings. And those nuns who evidenced positive attitudes about life and aging in their writings and in other testing were also much less likely to evidence the impact of dementia. Most people still associate the risk of Alzheimer's simply with age or with genetics, but the Nun Study revealed that it was learning and educational sophistication that would make the biggest difference in long-term cognitive health.

The researchers did have some surprises waiting for them when they cut open the nuns' brains. It turned out that some of the nuns possessed many of the physical manifestations of Alzheimer's—the tangles and plaques associated with dementia—but still exhibited normal cognitive functions in real life. Sister Esther, who lived to the age of 106, was known for her upbeat personality paired with an enthusiasm for books.[11] In her later years, she would give her exercise therapists yellow sticky notes with phrases from books she had read: "Think no evil, do no evil, hear no evil and you will never write a best-selling novel" was one such unlikely note she passed shortly before her death. In life, Sister Esther was energetic and cognitively intact, but her brain, when autopsied, was a mass of tangles. Snowdon chalked it up to Sister Esther's lifetime of learning and mental engagement which built cognitive reserve. In this way, the Nun Study essentially proved the importance of cognitive reserve—which Snowdon dubbed life's mental "spare tire"—to lifelong health and the fight against dementia.

Learning also plays a significant role in *physical* health, not just cognitive or mental health. It is in fact the case that the more education you have, the longer you will live and the healthier you will be. College graduates can expect to live about nine years longer than adults without a high school degree. We tend to think about health differentials as something that happens later in life, but in fact they show up throughout the life course: In rates of healthy live births, in rates of heart disease and diabetes, and even in drug use fatalities—and they favor those with more education at every stage. The bias is so strong that education levels extend through the generations. If you have lower educational achievements yourself, you pass on a life expectancy disadvantage to your children, even if they themselves end up among the better educated. And the correlation between health and education is not limited to, for instance, those with college degrees and those without; people with graduate degrees and

PhDs, for instance, are healthier than college graduates. Every year of education reduces your probability of death.[12]

This is mostly correlation. Education is connected with every-thing from higher income to better access to health care to lower stress and safer work and home environments. These are all incred-ibly important things to know about as concerned citizens, with significant implications about why people who lack formal educa-tional backgrounds are at a health disadvantage, but they probably are not relevant to decisions you will make about activities in the second half of life.

But there are causal factors as well. Educated adults have larger social networks—and these connections bring access to financial, psychological, and emotional resources that help reduce hardship and stress and improve health. The physical health benefits that flow from learning come less from what you know (though that matters) and more from the social and connective nature of the activity. Social engagement and connection are critical parts of the learning experience—at least with respect to in-person learning—and they have, as we have already seen, a direct and positive impact on long-term health.

The social aspect of learning is too often overlooked in an era of digital convenience. There are many advantages to digital learning: ubiquity, cost, and choice, not to mention the advantages for people with limited mobility. But virtual learning offers far less of the social connection that is so important to the learning experience, and lit-tle of the implied peer pressure that is a powerful outside motivator to staying engaged in learning. If we have discovered nothing else about education during the COVID-19 pandemic, it is that face-to-face learning is critical to socialization, to our sense of well-being and engagement, and to just feeling good and whole. In-person learning builds social capital,[13] and that is why Korea has continued to emphasize in-person adult education in support of healthy aging.

You can see that in the construct of learning programs. Two days before my trip to Changwon, I visited the Seoul Lifelong Learning Institute, an arm of the Seoul Metropolitan Government. I wanted to find out more about the extensive adult learning programming it provides across the sprawling city of 9.4 million people. They wanted to talk to me about Seventh Grade.

If you want to picture Seventh Grade, start with the image of students giggling and leaning into each other as they come off the last of the amusement park rides for the day. They are sure to be tired tonight, as it has been a long and exhausting day at the Seoul Children's Grand Park. Though these field trips are a lot for the teachers to manage, they are important rewards and a critical exercise in bonding and social cohesion among the students, none of whom knew each other before joining the class.

Not a terribly remarkable anecdote, you might be thinking, but undoubtedly others at the Children's Grand Park have taken surprised note of this group of seventh graders, because they are not your average pack of pimply-faced thirteen-year-olds. Instead, the students are all seventy years or older, the age requirement for participation in this particular seventh grade class.

The program, just launched in 2023, began with the observation that our early schooling years provide some of the strongest social connections, ties that often last a lifetime. And since one of the functions of the Lifelong Learning Institute is to help older adults not just learn but build the social connections that will sustain beyond the classroom, the theory went that the institute could incorporate the practices of grammar school into a new program for aging adults—and Seventh Grade was born.

The teachers of Seventh Grade have tried to preserve some of the cherished aspects of middle school—field trips, graduation ceremonies, even class officer elections (counterpoint from my teenage son, Nate: There are no cherished parts of middle school)—as a way of signaling that the social aspects of schools are as important as scholarly pursuits. But there are still classes in Seventh Grade, though they're a little different from the ones associated with middle school. Out goes biology and the dissecting of the fetal pig that I still remember with vague nausea almost fifty years on. In comes memoir writing, yoga, group therapy, and choir—including taking the choir on its own field trips to perform for outside audiences. But the core goal, the reason for wrapping the class in the trappings of long-ago schooling, is to create a new sense of belonging, community, and connection.

To be fair, my own recollections of seventh grade at Julius West Junior High are not all that fond, even discounting the fetal pig. I wasn't ever shoved in a locker, at least that my pride will let me remember, but the acrid taste of social flop sweat and romantic ineptitude lingers on many decades later. But it turns out that the students in their seventies make far more supportive and collegial classmates than the thirteen-year-olds of Rockville, Maryland. The director of the program, Kim Jong Sun, laughs when I ask her about this, and she assures me that an additional six decades of life have taken the edge off of school social competition.

Indeed, it is the social support and relationships that make Seventh Grade such an interesting program. It is now the highest-rated program in the institute's history, and the participants in Seventh

Grade have created their own ongoing social group, scheduling parties, cookouts, and trips together. Statistically reliable scientific data may not exist yet, but the participants think that the impact of the program on their health is clear. As one graduate reported, "After attending Seventh Grade, the number of trips that I have taken to the hospital has decreased. I feel happy and better."

It is a familiar refrain when you talk to people who are participating in adult classes in Korea. Older adults in Korea face a very specific struggle. With the traditional family structure at risk due to collapsing birth rates and the migration of younger people from secondary cities and rural areas to the Seoul Capital Region (which now boasts half of Korea's population), older adults struggle with chronic social isolation and resulting poor health. Classes like Seventh Grade are a lifeline for this population, which explains why so many people perceive such classes as having saved their lives.

———

The concept of a lifelong learning city was first developed in Europe as a project of the Organization for Economic Cooperation and Development (OECD), but progress in Europe has been sporadic, in part because communities often narrowly interpret the concept of lifelong learning cities as job training repackaged in a different form.[14] In contrast, Koreans have long viewed learning as a path toward personal enrichment and civic engagement and have made this type of learning a centerpiece of both national policy and personal identity.[15] Because of this, being deemed a "lifelong learning city" has become a point of community pride and a bit of a mania. Seoul is just one of about 170 Korean cities (out of a total of only 226 cities in the country) that have created lifelong learning institutes and have met the conditions to be designated as lifelong learning cities by the Ministry of Education.

Lifelong learning cities come in different flavors, but they all offer similar core services: hundreds of classes, typically free of cost, for adult education. The classes focus on personal enrichment, not marketable skills, so you won't find too many courses on Python programming or cybersecurity, but there are plenty on history, the humanities, music, Korean culture, art, and writing, for example. Lifelong learning centers occasionally offer digital courses, a practice that accelerated during the COVID-19 pandemic, but the vast majority of classes are in person, so as to foster community and social connections. Characteristically, classrooms are distributed throughout the city so that instruction is easier to access.

In Osan, the lifelong learning center is headquartered in a small strip-mall office with just enough space to house administrative offices and a couple classrooms. That's because most classes are parceled out across the city in what are called "stepping stone classrooms." There are 216 in all, and they are scattered across Osan in libraries, community centers, stores, and even teahouses. It's an astonishing number in a small city of roughly two hundred thousand, and it reflects the importance the city places on lifelong learning as it tries to help its citizens have engaged, productive, meaningful lives—and dissuade them from migrating twenty miles to the north to Seoul.

It's a challenge, though. Osan is a small city, overshadowed by the dynamism and scale of Seoul right next door. It does have a few points of civic pride: Osan is home to Korea's largest perfume and beauty products developer, Amore Pacific, and boasts one of the biggest markets in the country. The city was the site of the first clash between American and North Korean soldiers in the early days of the Korean War, and Osan Air Base, which houses a large American and South Korean military contingent, is named for the city, even though it is technically located outside the city limits five miles to the south. Beyond that, Osan doesn't have too much to brag about. Like much of Korea, Osan grew rapidly during the extraordinary economic expansion of the '80s and '90s without much regard to zoning, urban design, or architectural considerations. Dozens and dozens of featureless, matching apartment buildings, spread somewhat randomly around the city, both define and plague the skyline. Downtown, if you want to call it that, is home to a sea of squat, concrete block office buildings and a bewildering warren of shops and stores. It's Houston, without the charm.

That negative review of Osan is not shared by Park Ok Geum. Born in Daegu near the end of the Korean War, Park was raised in a working-class family that prized education. Unusual for girls of her time, she finished high school and aspired to be the first in her family to go to college. It was a goal shared, or at least not opposed, by her family, but reality intervened. Park never made it to college, instead remaining in the family home to help raise her younger siblings.

Her personal dream of college and learning never completely disappeared, but for thirty years it was buried deep beneath the responsibilities of family and work. She married, moved to Osan with her husband, and together they raised a family and ran a small grocery store. Finally, as her children went off on their own, and her clock ticked past age fifty, Park finally found the opportunity to start learning again. She had heard of what was then the fledgling Osan Lifelong Learning Institute and became one of its first students.

When she began taking courses, it was a whole new world: classes on recreation, laughter therapy, communications, and literature. She learned to play the guitar and the changgo, a traditional Korean drum—and performed for senior citizens. For more than a dozen years, Park took every class she could fit into her schedule, and she began putting to use what she was learning: teaching grammar and writing to elders who were not given the chance of a high school education in the postwar years. Park also volunteered as a "delivery teacher." When any five people in Osan get together and request a class on a specific topic, Osan Lifelong Learning provides a teacher and a classroom, and volunteer delivery teachers like Park are responsible for curriculum and content development.

Spending so much time in the Osan Lifelong Learning Program has opened up a new community and a new group of friends. Park told me that her "back is small, but [her] feet are wide." That may lose something in translation, but it reflects the fact that she has created a whole new base of support and social connective tissue that is sustaining her in good health.

Like so many I talk to, Park associates her experience with Osan Lifelong Learning with her improved health as she approaches seventy. Some of the connections are clear: Her class on laugh therapy has helped her relieve stress in a way that makes her feel materially better. Like so much associated with health, the broader picture is a little harder to define, yet Park is confident in her own personal health data. In that sense, Park is similar to so many people I met in Korea and elsewhere who celebrate the link between their flourishing health and being socially connected, not because of any research or doctor's opinion, but because they feel it in their hearts and in their own bodies. For Park, learning has given her a renewed sense of purpose, one that she worried would be gone with the closing of her shop and the maturation of her children. She tells me that this has translated to better health, including, in her view, her ability to recover from pancreatic disease. We'll never know of course whether she is specifically right about that, or whether a new treatment course, behavior change, or drug cocktail saved her life, but Park for one wants to give full credit to the value of learning and community.

As we talk, Park pulls out a photo album that she has compiled over the years, flipping through the pages to show me treasured memories. I see pictures of her playing the changgo, dressed in traditional Korean costume, and photos of her getting certificates of completion, all evidence of a life of commitment to learning and engagement. But the last picture is different. It's new, snapped just weeks before. It's a photo of Park in cap and gown, beaming as she receives her degree in lifetime education from Osan University. It was a prize denied her for a half century due to economic circumstances and cultural sexism and that has now been made possible because of the city of Osan's investment in lifelong learning. You might criticize the architecture in Osan, but in no way are you going to convince Park Ok Geum that Osan is not the best place on Earth.

Park has made learning her new career, but that takes planning. Maybe you (and the people of Table 23) are the rare individuals who can be productive, purposeful, and connected by taking it one day at a time, but that's not most people. Don't wake up at age sixty and expect a plan to unfold before you. That's the message that the Seoul city government is trying to send to its aging citizenry. The challenge of what to do with the second half of life is particularly acute in Seoul, a city in which millions of transplants are geographically divorced from family and where a competitive "up or out" business environment leaves many people in midlife unmoored from their work networks and a sense of purpose. It's a modern plague, one which Seoul pledged to combat with the launch of the Seoul 50 Plus Foundation a decade ago.[16] One of the key goals of the foundation is to help people in midlife, in their forties and fifties, fill in the "blank spaces" and engage in planning for what they want to do as they enter the next phase of life.

It's a remarkable turn: In the United States, we have seemingly endless resources for career and educational counseling for people in the first part of life, and any number of opportunities within companies or on the open market to help people plan out their careers. And there is a trillion-dollar retirement industry that is entirely focused on how to save money for retirement but has taken a hard pass on the question of what would make those years past the age of sixty healthy, productive, and purposeful.

In Seoul, however, you are not on your own. Although the idea for midlife renewal was pioneered at Seoul 50 Plus, the work is now shared with the city's Lifelong Learning Institute, which has created a Life Design course to help people in midlife imagine and plan for the second half of life. The curriculum for the course is a personal one; participants are encouraged to explore new topics, test new ideas, and imagine what their future might look like. Fundamentally, participants are encouraged to envision a wide-open future—to be more like Sarah and Jay than the people of Table 23—and they do, making plans to get degrees, begin volunteering, or even start a new business. I'm introduced to the story of one student who had invested years homeschooling his own children and had developed a personal expertise in Korean history. With his children grown, he was left at loose ends at the age of fifty-seven, lacking purpose and unsure of what to do next. He enrolled in the Life Design class and ultimately latched upon the idea of teaching Korean history to Korean children overseas, using Zoom to connect via a virtual classroom. These plans underscore the core idea of reinvention that is reflected in the Life Design School, as well as the Korean ideal that we never need to stop growing and learning.

Korea stands out, but a handful of other countries have also recognized the critical connection between lifelong learning and healthy longevity. In 2014, for instance, Singapore announced its multi-billion-dollar Action Plan for Successful Ageing and made lifelong learning a central component. At one level, it's not entirely surprising. Singapore has a bit of a national obsession with learning, dating all the way back to its post-independence strategies when education was seen as the key to economic development and societal stability.

With its Action Plan for Successful Ageing, Singapore launched two critical programs: the Skills Future program, which provides workforce training for every citizen in the country, and the National Silver Academy, which provides courses and learning opportunities for older citizens. Every citizen is eligible for an annual Skills Future credit (usable in either program), which makes adult education functionally free for virtually every Singaporean. The National Silver Academy provides access to a wide range of courses— from intellectual property law in Singapore to social-emotional learning and modern Tamil prose, to name just a few out of hundreds— but it's less the course offering and more the approach that stands out. At a time when more and more learning is moving online, the

National Silver Academy continues to emphasize in-person learning, even if it is for a digital literacy course, because of the critical social component it offers.

Older Americans like to learn too. According to the Pew Research Center, a hefty percentage, 62 percent to be exact, of Americans over the age of sixty-five identify themselves as lifelong learners,[17] an admirable number especially considering that only about a third of Americans have four-year college degrees. Independent of the level of education attainment, Americans think of themselves as learners and self-improvers, a nation of strivers: Almost 90 percent describe themselves as "looking for new opportunities to grow as a person." And if you ever want an advertisement for Wikipedia, just remember that 92 percent of adults agree with the statement that "I like to gather as much information as I can when I come across something that I am not familiar with." Older Americans correctly connect this with brain health: According to AARP, 83 percent of older Americans think it is vitally important to keep your brain active, and 68 percent think that life becomes stagnant without continuous learning.[18]

And there has never been a time in history when learning was more accessible. Online learning exploded during the COVID-19 pandemic, leaving Americans awash with learning options. There is the Khan Academy, Massive Online Open Courses (MOOCs) offered by universities or companies, ASU (Arizona State University) For You, and MasterClass, not to mention a nationwide community college system that offers a wide range of in-person and online classes. There's even an early-stage company called GetSetUp that is specifically focused on learning opportunities for people fifty-five and older. In combination, these services offer a diverse and occasionally weird range of content for older learners. At one point when I was writing this book, I logged on to GetSetUp and found opportunities to learn how to bake banana bread, remake old books into pieces of art, and practice chair yoga, kundalini style.

But even acknowledging GetSetUp and a few other similar enterprises, American adult learning is still overwhelmingly focused on the concept of career development. Americans have generally caught on to the fact that what you learn in high school and college may not be so relevant thirty years into your career when technology is being replaced every eighteen months. There are plenty of options, if not sources of funding support, to meet that need. But career development education generally ends with the career, leaving older Americans isolated from the educational process. The options that do exist for older Americans are perceived as elusive, expensive, and difficult to navigate. So not surprisingly, older Americans routinely identify costs, lack of time, and ageism as barriers to learning and in large numbers default to familiar and largely solitary activities like YouTube, magazines, and yelling at Rachel Maddow or Sean Hannity, depending upon your political preferences. That may sound ageist, and perhaps it is a bit, but these types of solitary engagements are by far the most frequently cited learning outlets for older Americans. Fuming along with the hosts at MSNBC about the latest Trump Administration outrage may offer a certain cathartic value, but it is unlikely to build the cognitive reserve that is critical to healthy aging.

Learning is healthiest when it is part of a collective, collaborative activity, but Americans learn alone. More than three-quarters of the people who identified themselves as lifelong learners told AARP that their principal means of learning was "reading on their own," an activity that would certainly have been embraced at Table 23, if not by social scientists.

———

The lifelong learning movement has adherents in all parts of the globe, even if efforts outside of places like Korea and Singapore tend to be limited in scope. Lebanon boasts of the University for Seniors, Japan has the Federation of Senior Citizens Clubs, and France can lay claim to the University of the Third Age (U3A), one of the first efforts to institutionalize learning for the over sixty set. U3A dates back to 1973, when the Faculty of Social Sciences in Toulouse, with support from the World Health Organization, the International Labour Organisation, and UNESCO, created a program to provide a permanent educational resource for older and retired people.[19] Despite its name, the U3A is not a university in the ordinary sense, but a loose confederation of volunteers working to create educational opportunities for later life and typically offering classes in topics ranging from movies to philosophy.

Over the last half century, the U3A model has spread beyond France, finding its strongest purchase in English-speaking countries like the UK, Canada, Australia, and Ireland. In the US, the torch of elder learning has been grasped most securely by the Osher Foundation, which has seeded Osher Lifelong Learning Institutes (OLLIs) at approximately 120 colleges and universities around the country.[20] The OLLIs offer noncredit courses, both online and in person, to people over the age of fifty, and they support a drop-in model that is typical of adult education in most parts of the world.

A small number of universities follow a more comprehensive residential model for older adults on a small scale. About forty fellows attend the Stanford Distinguished Careers Institute (DCI) each year, forking over the cost of a small home for the privilege of spending a year living the life of a Stanford undergraduate without the bother of grades or the peer pressure of fraternity rush.

Community colleges are also a key resource in the United States for lifelong learning. There are more than one thousand community colleges in the US with more than four million enrolled students at any one time. Admission is not quite open, but it is close: The then-chancellor of the California Community College system once bragged to me that his schools accepted the "top 100 percent of applicants." While various proposals to make community college free have stalled, tuition is still generally quite affordable, at least compared to four-year colleges, and many public community colleges provide free tuition to students over the age of sixty. Despite that, the prevalence of older learners is low. Community colleges specialize in nontraditional and older students, but typically that does not extend into later life. Only 8 percent of all community college students are over the age of forty, and most of them cluster toward the younger end of that range. This reflects our cultural bias against the idea of formal learning in retirement. When my friend (and contemporary) Charles posted on Facebook a picture of his first day of school at Pasadena City College, the common question from his online pals was about what he was teaching, not what he was taking (which was a digital photography class).

We should admire all these efforts, yet also acknowledge the limited impact they have had on a broader social level. Our culture has not kept up with the science of human connection, and our expectation of what later stages of life should be remains firmly moored in an early twentieth-century model. We live longer but increasingly in isolation from others around us. Even before COVID-19, time spent alone among Americans had increased substantially in the twenty-first century, with the heaviest burden falling on older Americans, who now report spending more than half of their waking time alone. But it is not just the old folks. In 2013, the average American reported spending six and a half hours a week with friends. By 2019, that number had declined to only four hours, an enormous decrease in just a few years.[21] That drop is almost certainly driven by technology, and it is unlikely that more technology is the solution.

———

Korea is a constant reminder of both the personal and the social value of a learning society. Back in Osan, I make a final stop at the Traditional Sunshine Tea House. It doubles as a stepping stone classroom, supervised by Lee Kyu Hee, who is billed to me as a tea master. It's a job title that even in modern-day Korea holds social currency, but Lee prefers to call herself an artisan of lifestyle and culture. Teahouses in Korea, like many traditional arts, are in a long-term secular decline, but the ones that remain, like Traditional Sunshine, are citadels of traditional culture and philosophy. Lee views her life's work as preserving the art of the tea ceremony and promoting a slower-paced way of life as a counterpoise to the hurry, hurry of modern Korea.

As part of the stepping stone network, Traditional Sunshine offers a course in the art of the traditional tea ceremony. The class typically runs for nine sessions and covers elements of Korean culture, as well as the traditions and forms of the tea ceremony. It also includes the preparation of traditional foods, with a special nod to the plain and healthy temple foods favored by Korean monks. I receive the accelerated version of the course—roughly one hour long—and we cover everything from the carefully orchestrated movements of the tea ceremony to the philosophies of Yi Hwang, a sixteenth-century Neo-Confucian scholar and a distant relation of Lee's. By the end of the hour, I am at once deeply gratified to have been exposed to such a diverse range of ideas and immensely relieved that I won't have to fold up my aching and shockingly inflexible legs under the low tea table for another eight hours.

Lee's class has proven immensely popular in Osan, but she noticed early on that enthusiasm for the teahouse course was concentrated among older Koreans. For Lee, who had started the course in part to share traditional Korean culture with younger people more familiar with Gangnam style than Gwon Geun styling,[22] this necessitated a rethink. And rethink it she did, as today you can walk out the door of Traditional Sunshine and within fifty paces bump into a new childcare and early education center, built to connect the youngest generation of Koreans with the oldest. Children from the center play in the yard of the teahouse and are also welcomed in for regular intergenerational events, such as a junior-sized tea ceremony held in collaboration with some of the area's elders. Sitting in Traditional Sunshine and talking with Lee, I can hear the children yelling and playing in exuberant voices not entirely suited to the serenity of the teahouse. I ask Lee how the children adapt to the manners of the teahouse (or perhaps how the teahouse accommodates children), and she laughs: "Outside they can be yelling and pushing, but inside, they immediately quiet down and sit quietly for the entire tea ceremony." The kids have fun, as do the seniors who more naturally gravitate to Traditional Sunshine.

It's not the only time that the stepping stone program brings the generations together. Each fall, Osan holds an annual Lifelong Learning Festival over the course of two weeks. All across the city, the stepping stone academies hold classes, open houses, and parties to highlight the importance and availability of lifelong learning. The event draws tens of thousands of people, a rather remarkable accomplishment in a city of a little more than two hundred thousand. It's remarkable but not unusual. The annual festival in Suncheon, held in the town's central park, is built around the theme of life's transitions and draws twenty thousand annually, roughly 10 percent of the population, while the lifelong learning festival held in the Gangnam district of Seoul dwarfs them all (though to be fair, everything in Seoul dwarfs the rest of the country), drawing more than a million people.[23] I've struggled to think of an analog in the US to the lifelong learning festivals held across Korea, and the nearest I can come are the state fairs held annually in forty-eight of the fifty states. Originally developed as agricultural and livestock exhibitions, the state fairs as a group have metastasized into something more eclectic: major concerts, roller coasters, and boardwalk games; something more weird: the great American duck race in Indiana and the five-hundred-pound butter cow carved annually for the Illinois State Fair; and something more fatty: the Texas State Fair's offering of some two hundred different types of fried food, including fried cheesecake and fried butter. And not to dismiss the connective value of both fried and deep-fried foods, but the cumulative differences between the lifelong learning festivals in Korea and the state fairs of the United States are as good of an explanation as any for the American life expectancy disadvantage.

Three Tips for Healthy Aging

The United States, along with the UK and Canada for that matter, is long overdue for an embrace of the idea of lifelong learning, and that may still develop as a logical corollary of an aging nation. But that's not happening today, and I for one don't want to wait around for a major policy shift.

Fortunately, there are already lots of opportunities out there if you know where to look. So here are three tips for lifelong learning:

Learn in person. There are many advantages to online learning: accessibility and choice chief among them. We all saw the value of online learning during the early days of the COVID-19 pandemic when use of adult learning platforms like Coursera boomed, rising by over 600 percent in some cases.[24] And there is no question that virtual learning can be a lifeline for people with disabilities or who otherwise have mobility restrictions. Let's praise virtual learning for what it brings but also acknowledge its limitations. Virtual learning lacks the social connections created by in-person learning, leading to reduced student satisfaction, boredom, loneliness, and depression.[25] And it lacks the stickiness of traditional in-person education. E-learning has long had a problem with high drop-out rates, and that is true for both adult learners and traditional school-age students.

If you can, take an in-person course. It's more effort, naturally, but that's part of the point. It gets you moving, tempts you out of the house, and most importantly, brings you into contact with all sorts of people. It's better both for learning and health.

Start early. Learning is not something that you should do early in life, abandon, and then pick up again at the last stages of life. Learning is a muscle that is best exercised at various stages throughout life. If you are in your forties or thirties or twenties, think of learning as a lifetime engagement, and plan what you might want to learn as you age—what is important now and what is likely to be most meaningful for you as you grow old.

It's never too late, though. I hope my mates at Table 23 will be inspired by the story of Park Ok Geum, who didn't return to school until her fifties—and then made a large personal commitment that transformed her life and her health. And I know others who didn't go back until their seventies and eighties. What connects this group is not the fact that they took a class—lots of people do that—but that they did it with a plan and a belief that this was part of a larger purpose for their later years.

Save your money. Americans identify money as one of the primary obstacles to lifelong learning in general, and late-life learning in particular. We're conditioned to think of learning as expensive, and with good reason. Tuition at public four-year colleges in the United States has increased by 750 percent since 1963, even after adjusting for inflation.[26] The good news is that there are extensive, though underpublicized, opportunities for seniors (usually defined for these purposes as people over the age of sixty) to attend school at steeply discounted prices. Virtually every state provides some form of tuition benefits for older adults at their public universities, colleges, and community colleges, and more often than not, the financial benefit is *free* tuition. The public universities in some states, like California, Connecticut, Louisiana, and Maine, waive tuition and most fees, including application fees. Other states, like Delaware, Utah, Virginia, Washington, Florida, and West Virginia, have laws requiring public institutions to provide free education to seniors. Georgia has, reminiscent of Korea, enshrined a right to free education for seniors in its constitution. Some states provide only a tuition reduction, though often a significant one; New Mexico charges the extravagant sum of five dollars per credit hour. And that's not even counting community colleges, many of which charge nothing to seniors. All this is to say that the opportunity for free or deeply discounted learning in an intergenerational setting is widely available. You only have to take advantage of it—and I hope Table 23 will.

Chapter 2

Bismarck's Revenge

E VEN AT AGE seventy-three, Yumiko Tankiwaki has no intention of slowing down. For the last eight years, she has worked part-time, three days a week, at the Kashiwa Pet Clinic in Fukuoka. It's a large clinic specializing in dogs and cats that employs five veterinarians and twice as many nurses, but on the day we visit, it has an empty, almost abandoned feel. The clinic is undergoing renovation, and all the cages are empty save for one that contains a lone, rather disoriented-looking cat. Without animals there's not too much to see, but that doesn't stop Tankiwaki from touring us around the office with evident pride. There are cages, lab equipment, a break room, a small surgery suite, and the world's tiniest elevator that seems suitable for a cat or a small dog but certainly not for the two fully grown humans that get stuffed inside.

It's understandable why she has such a proprietary feeling toward the clinic because in her estimation, the clinic has saved her life. Tankiwaki retired a decade ago, but when her husband died she felt adrift and alone, and her health declined. It's an all too familiar story on aging, that when the connective tissue of someone's life is

cut, whether it is to work or family, then bad health, even death, follows soon behind. Tankiwaki tells me how little meaning she could
find in her life without work or family. It left her depressed and
untethered, until she realized that many of her friends were finding
purposeful work through the Silver Jinzai Human Resources Center near them. She followed, signing up in the hope that working
would reduce her isolation and deep sense of loneliness. It worked.
With a big smile, she tells me that she "love[s] coming to work. . . .
The nurses are like my grandchildren, and working gives me purpose and has improved my health." It's a lovely story, almost making
up for that claustrophobic elevator, and now at seventy-three, she
has no plans to retire anytime soon—and neither do her friends,
all of whom continue to work into their mid-seventies and beyond.

Tankiwaki's story is a typical one. Across my travels in Japan, I
met dozens of older workers—in candy factories, machine shops,
car and bicycle parks—who told me of the central role of work in
creating purpose, meaning, and better health in their lives. Money
wasn't irrelevant to the conversation, it never really is, but it consistently faded into the background while meaning, purpose, and
vitality took center stage.

You can see that in the data from Silver Jinzai. In the mid-1970s,
aging advocates launched the Tokyo Metropolitan Senior Citizens
Corporation, designed to help older Japanese obtain part-time
work as a means of retaining vitality and health in retirement. In
the 1980s, the organization morphed into the Silver Jinzai Human
Resources Center, a government-supported entity that is now found
in virtually every community in the country. Silver Jinzai works
with businesses and workers to create jobs for older workers, all
part-time, in fields as diverse as park maintenance and agricultural

services. Over the years, the organization has become an important economic institution with almost seven hundred thousand registered seniors ranging in age from sixty to just about 100, the vast majority of them in the seventy and older age category and even 15 percent in the eighty and older category.[1]

And why do so many seniors register with Silver Jinzai? In a survey of new members in 2021, more than 80 percent reported that they signed up for Silver Jinzai for noneconomic reasons: to find meaning in life, to support social engagement, to meet new people, and to maintain and improve health.[2] It is essentially a consensus in Japan that work, purpose, and health are inextricably linked, and that concept is sometimes applied with rather startling specificity. When I visited the Ukiha no Takara company and finished my conversation with the three grandmothers, I talked with Mitsura Okuma, the local entrepreneur who had started the company. Okuma told me with confidence that my visit had added "three weeks" to the lifespan of the three grandmothers. I was a little surprised—all the evidence suggests that I am not a portable fountain of youth—and searched Mitsura's face to see whether it was a tongue-in-cheek comment. I couldn't tell for sure, but I don't think so, and instead the statement merely reflected his absolute faith in the link between work, social connection, and longevity.

The number of people sixty-five and older looking for work in Japan has doubled in the last decade,[3] and employment centers like Silver Jinzai and Hello Work are full of people saying things like "I'll be out of shape if I stay at home all the time, and the idea of stopping work completely makes me uneasy." But it's not full-time work they are looking for. Over half of all senior workers in Japan are classified as part-time workers, with less than a quarter working in full-time regular employment.[4] It's a new economy built to harness the needs and wants of older workers.

It's rather different in the West. In the US and the UK, and many other places in the West, work is more commonly associated with stress and ill health. A 2024 poll of workers in the US and the UK by Headspace, a company that provides employee mental health services, found that 77 percent of workers said stress at work contributed to negative health results.[5] And we commonly use language that associates work with poor health, even death. Who hasn't said something like "my boss is killing me," "this assignment will be the death of me," or "I'm killing myself to get my work done." It's not meant to be taken literally, but it reflects an underlying core belief that work diminishes our health and retirement liberates us.

———

I recognize that a chapter about why working longer is in our personal interest is not necessarily a crowd-pleaser. The cultural consensus in the West, and at Sarah and Jay's wedding, is that retirement is a natural right that begins as soon as possible, but generally no later than sixty-five. Attempts to reengineer the work and retirement system to support longer careers have been met with anger and defiance, even if the change is modest at best. In 2022, the plan of the Macron government in France to increase the mandatory retirement age from sixty-two to sixty-four generated an extraordinary outpouring of Gallic anguish. More than a million protesters took to the streets in January 2023, burning garbage cans, blocking roads, and generally bringing the country to a grinding halt. France is hardly alone. Tweaks to the retirement age in recent years have similarly brought angry crowds out to protest in countries as disparate as Greece, Morocco, and Kazakhstan, to name a few.

But this passionate adherence to the sanctity of the retirement age, whatever the specifics may be, is often of surprisingly recent vintage. In the 1960s in France, for instance, it was considered a "social death" to retire before sixty-five, and labor force participation rates by older workers were among the highest in the world. It wasn't until the election of the socialist government of François Mitterrand in 1982 that the retirement age was lowered to sixty, but that has not stopped the French from acting as though recalibrating it above sixty (or sixty-two, after it was revised upward in 2010) amounts to a functional death sentence for older people. That's not an exaggeration, as "metro, boulot, caveau" or "train, work, tomb" (a play on the French phrase "train, work, sleep" describing the daily grind) was a prominent protest statement during the strikes.[6]

It's all a little curious because retirement is hardly a paradise in France, with high rates of loneliness and social isolation among elders. But that's just a piece of it. Uproars over relatively small changes in the retirement age are rooted in the belief that there is something sacrosanct about age sixty-two or age sixty-five. But the fact that most countries group their retirement ages in the early to mid-sixties is largely an accident of history, the product of nineteenth-century Prussian politics rather than any careful study of physical capacity or the financial balance between work and retirement years.

The retirement age as we know it dates back to the late 1880s, when Otto von Bismarck, the long-serving chancellor of Germany, found himself in a precarious political position. Bismarck, known to history as the Iron Chancellor, had led Prussia through a tumultuous and transformative quarter century, a period in which Prussia gained preeminence within the German Federation, vanquished France, Austria, and Denmark in a string of wars, and spearheaded German unification. Even a century and a half on, it is still the case that there are few people who have had a larger impact on modern Europe than Bismarck, but by 1888, his political mastery was slipping. The young and ambitious new emperor, Kaiser Wilhelm II, thought Bismarck too old at age seventy-three and too cautious, and started making moves to sideline him. At the same time, an increasingly muscular and disruptive workers' movement, egged on by the socialists, was aggressively agitating for change. To appease the unions and create more maneuvering room for himself, Bismarck proposed a series of new labor laws and social reforms, including the continent's first public pension plan.

Bismarck's plan was unprecedented in modern European history—until then, the very concept of a pension was unknown: You worked until you died, and your grave was your retirement plan. Even dangling the idea of a pension must have been exhilarating, as it promised the prospect of financial security for workers who too often faced terrible conditions and exploitative financial arrangements. But Bismarck was no friend of the working man. He set the age for pension eligibility at seventy (subsequently shaved down to sixty-five) at a time when life expectancy in Germany was only forty-three. It was thin gruel to be sure, but it did provide one of the first steps, however tentative, toward the modern European pension system.

Alas, Bismarck's political craftsmanship was not enough to save his job, and he was forced out by Kaiser Wilhelm in 1890. Showered with titles that included the Duke of Lauenburg and

"Colonel-General with the Dignity of Field Marshal" for the German Army, Bismarck had the secure retirement that eluded the
mine and factory workers of Germany. But he also left behind a
program that had the unexpected consequence of enshrining the
idea of retirement in the public's mind and eventually fixing the
consensus retirement age at sixty-five. Decades later, FDR and his
reformers latched on to that number and made it a lynchpin of
the new American Social Security laws. Now, more than 130 years
later—after adding thirty-five to forty additional years to average
life—the number picked by Bismarck to evade broad financial lia-
bility remains the standard date for retirement in most of the developed world.[7]

In most of the world, retirement practices remain oddly divorced
from underlying economics and government policy. In the 1950s in
the United States, the average retirement age was 68.7, even though
the life expectancy for an American man was only 65.6. You do the
math. There were a decent number of people who beat the actuarial roulette wheel and made it to retirement, of course. That group
could do all of the things culturally associated with the retirement
years—bouncing grandchildren on the knee, puttering in the garden, and taking long walks on the beach—just so long as the walks
weren't too long. Since then, even as life expectancy has added more
than a decade to life and as Social Security policy has increased the
date of full eligibility to sixty-seven (and provided additional incentives to delay to age seventy), the actual retirement age of Americans has declined, now landing close to sixty-two.[8] Some of this is
driven by the very real difficulties older workers face in retaining a
job or finding new work, but part is driven by a shared notion that
ending work is the goal. I'd call it very French in attitude, though

many American and British workers would likely resent that, but there is a common assumption across many cultures that life is better in the absence of work.

———

Even though the very concept of retirement is relatively new, we now view it largely as a right, the logical culmination of the three-stage step from education to work to retirement. But it's not that way in Japan. There, you will find an entirely different attitude about working longer, not because the government has changed retirement rules (though it has), but because of social attitudes and the philosophy of life known as ikigai.

Just before I left for Asia, I visited with Bradley Schurman, the author of the book *The Super Age* and a noted expert on longevity.[9] It's often hard to book interviews from ten thousand miles away, especially when there are language barriers to overcome, and Bradley, who has traveled extensively in Asia, had been making introductions for me in Japan and Korea. Over drinks, he offered me all sorts of useful travel advice, from how to navigate the Tokyo subway (though nothing can really prepare you for that) to the best time to visit the fish markets in Seoul (very, very early). Just before we parted, Bradley reached into his bag and handed me a book titled *Ikigai: The Japanese Secret to a Long and Happy Life*, written, curiously enough, by two Spaniards, Héctor García and Francesc Miralles.[10] I had a long list of books I wanted to read before I reached Korea, my first stop, and I was tempted to shove *Ikigai* to the bottom of the pile, but it had the attractive quality of being short, so it ended up on the top of my stack.

It's a good thing too, because people in Japan talk about ikigai all the time. It's a little startling. I've traveled all over the US and talked with hundreds of workers about their jobs and their retirement. Book interviews, podcast interviews, focus groups, lots of random conversations in Ubers, airports, and coffee shops—and not once has anyone mentioned a philosophy of life, of any type. But in Japan, everyone knows ikigai, and at least half the older workers I interviewed mentioned it in some fashion. And even among those who didn't say the word "ikigai" by name, many expressed a belief in the "happiness of always being busy," which is a pretty fair summary of what ikigai is all about.

Ikigai is composed of two words: *iki*, which means life, and *gai*, which describes value or worth. In the West, it is often depicted as a Venn diagram with four overlapping qualities: what you love, what you are good at, what the world needs, and what you can be paid for. Within Japanese culture, the concept of ikigai relates to the effort to find joy in everyday tasks, to take pleasure from completing a task, or the satisfaction from an interchange with a friend, a colleague, or a customer. The psychiatrist Mieko Kamiya has put it this way: "Japanese people believe that the sum of small joys in everyday life results in more fulfilling life as a whole."

One important element of ikigai is microflow, taking joy in the simplest of tasks. Psychologist Mihaly Csikszentmihalyi defines the concept of flow as "the state in which people are so involved in an activity that nothing else seems to matter; the experience itself is so enjoyable that people will do it at great cost, for the sheer sake of doing it." Microflow means finding value in even mundane tasks, concentrating on one task at a time, and discovering the joy of simplicity and attention to detail. It's an important concept in Japan because much of the work assigned to older people is often of the rote variety, but the value of the work comes not from the prestige, but from the simplicity of doing it well.

Work is not the only source of ikigai, but increasingly it is seen as *the* way for older Japanese to find ongoing purpose. Even given the tremendous social respect afforded older Japanese, the years past sixty-five can be challenging ones, filled with increasing risks of social isolation. Japan may be the longest-lived and healthiest country on Earth, but it has not been immune from the modern ills of loneliness. The severance of relationships at work, growing physical distance from grown children, and the dispersal (and yes, death) of friends and peers all create risks of social isolation and loss of the sense of belonging. For older Japanese, it is commonly understood that work is a haven from these challenges, a place to find meaning, create social connection, and retain their place in the cultural universe.

Ikigai is by no means a new concept, though it gained broader public awareness and popularity with Kamiya's writings in the 1960s. But it began to substantially influence the relationship between older people and work in the last three decades. Historically, Japan maintained a very rigid retirement system, with most companies requiring retirement by age sixty-five in order to make way for younger workers and reduce the heavy financial carrying cost sometimes associated with older employees. But at the turn of the century, a number of factors came together to revolutionize the Japanese employment system. Older adults became more physically capable, and they increasingly perceived work as a key mechanism to stay active and healthy. And Japanese companies, faced with declines in the pool of workers aged eighteen to sixty-five, in turn started to see older workers as critical components of the labor force. As a result, Japan developed a system of "reemployment" that brought back retired workers on lower-cost contracts right after retirement, and companies began to develop flexible work opportunities designed to attract and retain older workers. In a matter of years, Japan evolved from one of the most rigid and inhospitable employment systems for older workers to one of the most inviting.[11]

You can see that evolution at Yamada Kogyo, a producer of specialized heavy equipment in Toyama, a mid-sized city on the west coast of Japan. Hiro and I don hard hats and enter a cavernous, poorly lit fabrication plant. Even in an increasingly mechanized world, the shop floor reeks of hard manual labor: Blowtorches sparkle and metal-on-metal sounds echo across the gloomy room. It's not a place where you would expect to find older workers, and until relatively recently that was true, as the company enforced a strict retirement age of sixty. But Toyama, and Yamada Kogyo, sit on a demographic cliff. The Japanese workforce in general is aging rapidly, but the problem is particularly acute in secondary cities like Toyama. Despite its obvious appeal—the beautiful mountains, its beckoning shoreline, and the fairy-tale castle plunked right in the middle of town—young people are increasingly fleeing mid-sized cities like Toyama, lured away by the delights and better job opportunities in Tokyo and Osaka. Keiko Yamada, the company's CEO, had inherited a rigid work environment that served her father well but no longer made sense for the company. With younger workers disappearing and an aging labor force possessing key institutional knowledge of how their tools are designed and fabricated, Keiko Yamada knew that change was both inevitable and necessary.

Out went long-standing retirement rules and age restrictions on labor, and in came a flexible set of rules to support older workers. As we walk the plant floor, I can see that the workforce is now full of people, almost all men, in their sixties, seventies, and even approaching eighty. As I talk with the workers, they say many of the things that I hear across Japan: They work to give themselves a purpose in life, to ward off the loneliness of later life, and to make sure that they stay active, healthy, and socially connected. And when I ask them how long they intend to work, they say, as so many others have said to me, "Until I can't." If there was going to be a song about the goals of older workers in Japan, "Until I Can't" would be the title, because it so well captures the cultural consensus in Japan that work is intrinsic to purpose, to health, and should end only when one's individual situation requires it, and not at some arbitrary pre-designated date.

But "until I can't" wouldn't be possible without the change to work rules. I chat with two older workers who jointly manage the cost and accounting systems for the company. They both work three days a week, and they start an hour later than other workers on those days. Their schedule is replicated for older workers on the shop floor. All of this would have been unthinkable when Keiko Yamada's father ran the company, but it is an increasingly common arrangement in this super-aged nation.

———

At one level, it makes sense that Japan, as the world's oldest nation, is at the forefront of change, but in other ways, it is an unlikely revolutionary. Work in Japan has long been a high-stress environment with a rigid and conformist set of rules. And for many workers, that hasn't changed. Over half of Japanese workers report being stressed at work, with the amount of work being the most significant source of this stress.[12] Seventy-three percent of Japanese workers have told Gallup that they are not engaged in their work, compared to the global average of 59 percent. And rates of suicide and mental health challenges remain troublingly and intractably high for Japanese workers as a whole.[13]

But it's not that way for older workers because they hold the high cards in Japan. Japanese companies need them more than they need the jobs, and that has compelled many Japanese companies, long renowned for their inflexible and uniform approaches to work rules, to adapt to the different needs of older workers. Nearly 40 percent of companies in Japan now hire workers past age seventy,[14] and the vast majority of these businesses have launched new programs to attract and retain older workers. In addition to flexible hours and part-time work, companies like Konica Minolta and Canon have implemented career design programs to support mid-career workers in planning and training for longer careers. Other companies, such as skincare manufacturer FANCL and air-conditioning producer Daikin, have revamped their pay and benefits programs to encourage workers to extend past traditional retirement age.[15] And the Japanese government has pitched in as well, offering subsidies to companies that are hiring older workers and promising an investment of one trillion yen (roughly equivalent to 6.5 billion US dollars) over five years to support retraining and reskilling. It's an entire work ecosystem being built to support older workers, but it would not be sufficient unless older Japanese workers saw the connection between continued employment, purpose, and good health.

———

Echoing general societal beliefs, employers in many parts of the world perceive older workers as slower, less technology-savvy, and out of touch. It's reflected in our culture: Think of Creed in *The Office*, Mr. Burns in *The Simpsons*, President Biden in the White House. We live in ageist societies, and that is perhaps felt most dramatically in the workplace. In the United States, two-thirds of companies view older employees as putting them at a competitive disadvantage, so it is no surprise that a full 75 percent of workers over the age of fifty report experiencing or witnessing ageism in their workplace. Older workers are most likely the first to be let go and the last to be hired back. It's not even really a secret, even though age discrimination against workers over the age of forty has been illegal in the US since the passage of the Age Discrimination in Employment Act in 1967. I once had a senior executive at United Airlines ask me if I had any expertise in *getting rid* of older workers, and she was visibly disappointed when I broke it to her that I was more interested in how to keep them.

The issue is particularly acute in industries like technology and media that help drive cultural norms. Mark Zuckerberg famously said, at the tender age of twenty-three, that "young people are just smarter," though perhaps he has reconsidered that view now that he is north of forty. But whether he has revised his views in light of his own age or not, the cult of youth permeates the industry. Silicon Valley boasts one of the greatest concentrations of Botox clinics and plastic surgery shops in the world, because the young tech engineers and entrepreneurs who frequent them believe that they would be at a competitive disadvantage if they are perceived as too old.[16] And for good reason: Many Silicon Valley investors have a rough guideline of never investing in a start-up led by anyone over the age of thirty-two, even though older entrepreneurs are the fastest-growing category in the country, and older founders outperform the marketplace.[17]

It's not just high-end jobs. To test ageist practices in hiring, researchers at the University of California, Irvine, and Tulane University submitted forty thousand résumés in response to ads for jobs that employ large numbers of low-skilled workers of all ages, such as administrative assistants, janitors, security guards, and retail sales. The résumés were evenly distributed between young (ages twenty-nine to thirty-one), middle-aged (forty-nine to fifty-one), and older (sixty-four to sixty-six) and were functionally equivalent but for the age of the fictional applicants. The younger workers fared best, garnering far more interviews than the oldest applicants, especially older women.[18] For the sales position, younger women scored 60 percent more interviews than the older women, even though they had the same qualifications.

Even in some of the tightest labor markets in decades, American companies can't wrap their heads around the fact that older workers are a growing and critical source of talent. In an era in which diversity, equity, and inclusion has become a buzzword at every major company (and now runs the risk of becoming a swear word), it is shocking how few companies consider age diversity. Only 8 percent of companies report that age is part of their diversity goals, and even among that 8 percent you have to look awfully hard to find any serious efforts to accommodate the needs of older workers. CVS has a "snowbird" program, allowing older pharmacists to work at stores in the south during the winter,[19] and both B&Q, the British home supply store, and Home Depot, its American counterpart, have affinities for older workers because they think shoppers want to "ask their fathers" for home improvement advice, but they are the exception, even as companies report labor shortages and hiring shortfalls.

———

The health effects of work versus retirement have been studied extensively, with research projects conducted across the US, Europe, and the advanced economies of Asia. It's a hard issue to study because it is difficult to isolate the impact of work from all the other factors that affect our health as we age. Difficult, though not impossible, and over the last decade, the evidence has emerged that work in later life is beneficial to your long-term health and that it is one of the key antidotes to loneliness, isolation, and the negative health consequences that typically follow.

You can see that in the results of the Harvard Study of Adult Development. People who have strong social relationships at work, especially those who can identify a "best friend" on the job, and those who can identify a positive purpose in their work, are happier and healthier and live longer than similarly situated people who don't. Other studies have shown similar large-scale effects over time for older adults. A study that tracked eighty-three thousand older adults over the course of fifteen years, published in the Centers for Disease Control and Prevention's journal *Preventing Chronic Disease*, found that compared with people who retired, those who worked past the traditional retirement age of sixty-five were three times more likely to report being in good health. They were also about half as likely to have serious health problems such as cancer or heart disease.[20]

But there is a potential bias to the data that could skew those results. Since some people leave the workforce simply because they are unhealthy, you might expect workers to be healthier than non-workers for reasons that have nothing to do with the health impact of work. In recent years, though, researchers have begun to deal with this "healthy worker" effect. In 2016, a team from Oregon State University conducted a study of three thousand American workers and retirees over the age of sixty-five. They categorized workers as either healthy or unhealthy and analyzed each group separately. Even after this sorting process, the research team found that working past the traditional retirement date still helped older adults maintain social connections and a sense of purpose, thereby delaying the cognitive and physical declines typically associated with aging. And this held true across both healthy and unhealthy groups, and across a wide range of sociodemographic, lifestyle, and health-related conditions. Working even one more year beyond the typical retirement age reduced the risk of mortality by about 10 percent during the eighteen-year period of the study, regardless of your health. Other studies in Greece, Austria, Sweden, the US, and Germany have reached similar results.[21]

We tend to think first of the impact of work on physical health. It makes sense. Work, at least in-person work, requires extensive physical activity even for deskbound jobs. When you're young, you might not even classify the effort to get from home to work and back again as physical activity, but even getting out of the home, commuting to work, and all the intrinsic activities associated even with office work form an important physical distinction between work and retirement. But the impact of work on cognitive health is at least as important.[22] Large-scale studies in both Sweden and China have associated retirement with increased risk of dementia and cognitive decline.[23] The Chinese study is particularly revealing because the researchers found that in their study group, the pensioners ate more healthfully, slept more, and drank less, yet they fared materially worse than the workers when it came to measures of cognitive decline. You can exercise all you want, get those solid eight hours of sleep, and just churn through all those avocados and dark chocolate or whatever superfoods you prefer, but if you don't have the social engagement that is intrinsically associated with work, your cognitive health could still suffer. This is not to say that there aren't jobs that are dull or unrewarding—only about 40 percent of American workers describe their jobs as "good"[24]—but even the vast majority of poor or fair jobs involve customer or colleague interactions that have proven to be more mentally stimulating than the cognitive idleness of most retirements.[25]

Despite the evidence, we continue to undervalue the connection between work and social health. We view retirement as a relief from work, a way to reduce stress in our lives. But that ignores the stress of loneliness and isolation that often comes with retirement, leading to sometimes dramatic and unpleasant consequences. As the US Surgeon General's Report on the Loneliness Crisis puts it: "[f]or people who are lonely and isolated, there is no return. They live in a state of constant stress, to their physical detriment."

You can see why retirement, with the almost invariable retreat from long-standing social networks, raises significant health challenges. Yet, in popular lore, retirement, especially the first decade of it, is depicted as a time of health, vigor, and leisure, a time to regain personal equilibrium after the stress of work. Google "what is retirement like" and you will get inundated with images of happy couples—almost always couples—tracing hearts on the beach, enjoying beautiful views from matching Adirondack chairs, or riding tandem on Jet Skis or mopeds, arms stretched into the air with joy. Retirement is blissful, stress-free, and apparently involves just endless amounts of paired, unsafe transportation.

The reality for most people is rather different. Narrowing social networks as people lose work connections, constrained financial situations, loss of purpose, and declining mobility as people find less and less reason to leave the house are all characteristics of even the early years of retirement. And reduced health often follows. According to some of the largest studies of health panels across Europe, retirement leads to a worse health trajectory, with decreases in the likelihood of being in "excellent" or "very good" self-assessed health by 39 percent, increases in clinical depression by 41 percent, increases in chronic conditions by 63 percent, and 60 percent increases in the likelihood of needing to take a drug to manage health.[26] There are all sorts of unintended and frankly unhappy results associated with retirement that you may want to think through. During the conflict in France over raising the retirement age, protesters held aloft signs saying, "I need time for sex," but they had it exactly wrong. Sex drops off dramatically after retirement because loneliness, lack of purpose, and too much time on your hands are apparently not aphrodisiacs. Your results may vary but suffice it to say that if you want to maximize your odds of a longer, healthier life, you will, like so many of the Japanese workers who I talked to, want to keep working as long as you can.

——

And how long you can is likely a lot longer than it used to be, a fact I see virtually from the moment I step foot into Japan. I arrive by boat, taking the ferry from Busan in Korea to Fukuoka on the southern island of Kyushu. I'm not much of a seafarer, as my occasional green coloring can attest, but I was charmed by the idea of arriving by sea. I imagined myself straddling the deck, wind whipping my hair (in my imagination, I still have hair), peering through the mists as the shoreline of Kyushu emerged. Alas, the reality is less romantic. The JR Beetle is a hydrofoil with no accessible deck space and large signs in Korean, Japanese, and English forbidding customers from whipping their hair in any way. I settle instead for watching *Indiana Jones and the Dial of Destiny* in Korean on the small, shared television hanging from the ceiling a few rows in front of me. But as it turns out, a movie in which an eighty-year-old Harrison Ford plays a train-jumping, fist-throwing, gun-toting, time-traveling action star is an appropriate introduction to Japan.

The next morning is Sunday, so I have tourist time, and I head for Tochoji Temple. Built in 806 CE, the original temple burned down, as things in Japan tend to do, and was rebuilt on its current spot in the late sixteenth century. It is one of the oldest and most famous Buddhist temples in Japan, but despite its venerable age, its most notable feature, the one that makes all the tourist books, is of relatively new vintage: an eleven-meter, thirty-ton statue of the Buddha that was built over four years starting in 1992. It's the largest wooden-seated Buddha in all of Japan, which is a very specific claim to greatness, but I'm a complete sucker for the largest of most anything.

It's a bit of a busman's holiday for me. Even on the short walk to Tochoji Temple, it's impossible for me to ignore the extraordinary number of older people on the street. Fukuoka, by Japanese standards, has a relatively young population, but it's very old compared to everywhere else: Just under 30 percent of the city's population is over the age of sixty-five, compared to 17 percent and 19 percent in the US and the UK, respectively. You can see the age of people in their faces, but you might not know it otherwise. The older pedestrians easily keep pace with the younger ones, and canes, walkers, and wheelchairs are virtually nonexistent. The only concession to age that I can observe is that the countdowns on the crosswalks are extended to give older folks more time to get across the street, but I'm not actually sure that they need it.

You don't need to take my word for it. For generations, social scientists have been tracking the walking speeds of different age cohorts in Japan to chart the physical progress of older people and assess whether there have been improvements (or declines) over the years. There are many measures of physical performance, but walking speed is considered to be a particularly important one because it is the best measure of mobility, a critical function for older adults hoping to live on their own. In older people, declines in walking speed are known to be a predictive factor for risk of falling, depression, admission to a health care institution, cognitive decline, and even death.[27]

Over the last thirty years, the walking speeds of older Japanese men and women have been increasing at staggering rates. The average walking speed of both men and women in their early eighties today is now higher than for sixty-five to sixty-nine-year-olds in 1992. In fact, the foot speed of people *over the age of eighty-five* is now almost equivalent to that of people in their late sixties in 1992, and women eighty-five and older are now significantly faster than women fifteen years younger were in the early 1990s. In every way, older Japanese, especially women, are far healthier, stronger, more mobile, and more active than fellow Japanese of the same age just

one generation ago. We are accustomed by now to anodyne statements like "seventy is the new fifty," and they have always struck me
as more self-aggrandizing than anything else, but as it turns out, for
the Japanese, it's scientific fact. The biological clock for many people
here in Fukuoka may read eighty or ninety, but it is the case that
they are far more physically capable than their parents' generation
even when they were ten or fifteen years younger.[28]

And it's not just walking speeds. In just the last decade, grip
strength, another all-purpose measure of physical capacity in older
people, has increased substantially for almost all older age groups
in Japan. Collectively, these studies of older people in Japan paint
a picture, one that I see on the streets of Fukuoka, of a far more
physically fit and physically capable population, one that is being
described as a rejuvenated generation of "young old people." They
may not all be quite ready to wrestle Nazi villains on top of moving
trains, a la Indiana Jones, but they are getting closer.

There are multiple reasons for the physical rejuvenation of older
Japanese. Diet likely plays a role in this, though perhaps not what
you think. In the West, the Japanese diet, with some good reason, is
lauded for its use of fresh vegetables and rice, but it is the increase in
animal protein that is most often cited as the reason for the increase
in height, weight, and strength among older Japanese in recent
years. And increasingly scientists point to the increase in social participation that has reduced the risk of functional disability, decline,
and depressive symptoms.[29]

It is indisputably true that physical capacities wane in later life,
but our assumptions about when and how much that happens are
far out of date. Our cultural clock remains frozen in the middle of
the last century, fixed on the notion that sixty or sixty-five is the

beginning of some irredeemable period of infirmity and decline—a period in which "I'm too old to work" becomes a defining characteristic of our lives.[30] I'm not sure when "old age" begins, and I'm not even sure that the question makes much sense given the increasing physical and cognitive heterogeneity of people as they age. But it is clear to me that these rules we have about retirement, developed in a bygone epoch and reaffirmed in a period when our age clock was entirely different, are not only out of whack with our economic needs as a society, but also our own personal needs to age well.

———

I reach down, grasp the basket, and straighten up. The basket is heavy—it contains about twenty kilograms of barbells—and I grunt audibly as I finish the motion and then repeat the task an additional four times. Hiroshi, the designer of the exoskeleton suit I just strapped on, reaches over and activates it, inviting me now to repeat the task with the assistance of the "muscle suit." I'm not terribly eager to continue the weightlifting course, but I'm curious about the impact of wearing the exoskeleton. I pick up the basket again: It's not light as a feather, it's still fifty or so pounds, but the task of lifting and moving the basket is now much, much easier. No grunting required.

The Hiroshi in this story is Hiroshi Kobayashi, a professor of mechanical engineering at the Tokyo University of Science and the inventor of the muscle suit, an exoskeleton that relies on compressed air technology to relieve pressure on the back and assist workers with heavy, repetitive tasks. Originally, Kobayashi developed the muscle suit with the hopes of helping disabled people and patients in nursing homes, but it didn't quite catch on, as it couldn't help

with the mobility challenges most significant to that group. Nonetheless, word seeped out about his invention, and Kobayashi started
hearing from companies who thought that the muscle suit could
help their employees. Many companies in Japan were struggling, he
was told, with the challenge of extending the working life of their
aging workforce, and the muscle suit responded to that need perfectly by reducing wear and tear and making physical work easier.
If provided to younger workers, the muscle suit would allow them
to work longer with greater ease, and if provided to older workers,
it would help them do physical tasks they might not otherwise be
able to perform.

Ten years ago, Kobayashi launched a company called Innophys
to further develop and market the muscle suit.[31] Today, it's used by
some ten thousand companies, mostly in Japan but also in twenty-
plus other countries. That list does not include the United States
because the current design does not conform—Hiroshi dances
around it but finally admits it—to the larger (and growing) girth of
the average American worker.

The muscle suit is marketed to and used by workers of all
ages, but it has particular appeal to older workers. I've described
the remarkable physical progress of older Japanese, but they're not
invincible. Older workers almost always lose strength and flexibility, but the muscle suit reduces the impact of physical decline,
extending work life and allowing more older workers to remain
active in the labor force. When I picture the primary use case for
the muscle suit, I invariably think of workers in a warehouse, load-
ing and unloading heavy boxes. Hiroshi tells me, though, that the
muscle suit has proven particularly popular with Japanese farmers.
Agriculture plays a significant role in Japanese culture, but in an era

of urbanization and worker scarcity, life on the farm has not proven appealing to younger Japanese workers. That has left a significantly older farm worker population, one dedicated to preserving heritage farming in Japan but increasingly pressed to meet the significant physical challenges of the job.

The muscle suit is not the only technology used by older farmers. In Toyama, I meet Keiko Inada, the general manager of Sky Intec, a large national IT consulting firm. Toyama has long cultivated an image as an age-friendly city, investing heavily in everything from age-accessible transportation to thermal baths that are believed to be healing for older people. Work is a part of the strategy—the city has bought a lot of muscle suits—and the city government has lobbied employers to find ways to support older workers, especially in the agricultural sector. Sky Intec is not a natural fit for agricultural innovation, but like many Japanese companies, it is trying to do its part by using technology expertise to build solutions for older farmers. The company's engineers have built a robot to accompany farmers in the field and ferry crops back to their warehouses, saving farmers the wear and tear of carrying the harvest back themselves. The robot, which looks a little bit like a low-slung dog, has overcome the challenge of navigating rough terrain filled with furrows, plants, and other obstacles with sufficient reliability to be a useful companion for farmers. The company has even gone as far as to buy up farms and arrange for the farmers to continue to work them so as to relieve the older farmers of many of the administrative hassles and uncertainties that come with running a small family business. In the process, Sky Intec has become the nation's largest grower of Nashi pears—a very odd distinction for a tech company. In the US, such an arrangement would certainly raise eyebrows about strategy and focus and perhaps even suspicions about the exploitation of older farmers, but in Japan it makes complete sense in the context of society's support for older workers.

Throughout Japan, companies, organizations, and individuals are deploying new technologies to extend careers and make work practical for older workers. Some of it is assistive technology like the muscle suit; some of it helps older workers have more flexible work environments, like the artificial intelligence systems being developed to support job-matching and job-sharing arrangements. All of this has contributed to soaring employment rates for older Japanese workers. In 2022, there were 9.1 million workers above the age of sixty-five in Japan, a number that has increased for nineteen straight years and is almost double what it was just a dozen years ago. More than half of all people in Japan between the ages of sixty-five and sixty-nine are employed, over a third between the ages of seventy and seventy-four are still working, and even 11 percent of people over the age of seventy-five have jobs. It's a revolution in the scope of work and the meaning of retirement.[32]

———

Older workers are of course not evenly distributed across the economy. They cluster in jobs that allow for flexibility and human connection. Everywhere I turn in Asia, my cab or Uber driver is older than me, sometimes significantly so. It starts right away when my airport train deposits me at Seoul Station, one of the central hubs in the city. I'm tired after a long flight and looking forward to crashing at my Airbnb apartment in the Itaewon section of town. The cab line pairs me with a driver who is seventy-five if he is a day, and we reach our first cultural impasse. Welcome to Seoul. He doesn't speak English. I don't speak Korean, and my phonetic pronunciation of the address, along with frantic jabs at the map on my phone, is not getting it done. We are both frustrated, as tired travelers and drivers sometimes get, and in an earlier day, that might have ended our brief business relationship. But today my cabbie has access to an over-the-phone translation service. In a couple minutes, we are on our way: me still skeptical but willing to suspend disbelief because what choice do I have, and him driving with a confidence, speed, and urban arrogance that would have the pride of any New York City driver (or Hell's Angel biker, for that matter). Fifteen minutes later, he deposits me in front of a Korean "Friend" Chicken outlet that is, to my happy astonishment, right below my Airbnb apartment.

There is something about cab drivers that puts them on the front lines of the debate around older workers. In New York City, the median age of a cab driver is only forty-six. In Paris it's forty-eight, and in London it's fifty. But in Tokyo, the average age is fifty-eight, and seven out of ten taxi drivers in Seoul are in their sixties or seventies.[33] In Singapore, the government has gradually raised the retirement age of cab drivers, first from seventy to seventy-three in 2006 and then to seventy-five in 2012.[34] In Japan, the government has already announced plans to raise the retirement age to eighty, though many cab drivers are already over that age due to the way the law is structured.[35] Korea has no driver retirement age at all.

If that makes you nervous, you're better off staying at home. In the West, we associate older drivers with danger, driving too slow, and poor reaction times. It's the grandmother peeking over the steering wheel and the grandchildren arguing about when to take away the keys. But in the long-lived Asian societies, older age is more commonly associated with better judgment and greater experience, while youth is associated with recklessness and poor driving habits, a view borne out in general driving data. When it comes to cab drivers, the comparisons are less clear; the best existing study on cab driver safety suggests that older drivers have greater work efficiency and work quality but compare unfavorably when it comes to adherence to traffic laws, and I suspect my first driver that day in Seoul is Exhibit A for that problem.[36]

It's not just Seoul. In Busan, my cabbie is a tiny woman in her seventies. She takes me on after three other cabbies turn me down, leaving me a bit pissed off at the cab industry and the whole city of Busan for good measure. I don't know that my fourth cabbie understands me any better than the others, but maybe she is just more game than the rest. She works through the various Google maps to get me to my hotel, or to be fair, to get me close enough to it that I can hoof the last two blocks.

Korea is jam-packed with older workers, rivaling and perhaps exceeding Japan, depending upon what dataset you reference. The reasons for working later in life in Korea are more varied and complicated than those in Japan, and they often include the economics of a country without a strong social safety net and where many older people missed out on the financial windfall of the Korean economic miracle. But work is also a growing source of social connection and purpose in a country where the multigenerational family as the central social unit is decaying due to plunging birth rates and urbanization.

There are older working people everywhere in Seoul. The average age of retirement from a first career in Korea is only forty-nine, so much of the workforce is working on a second or third career.

But even in Seoul, a city used to older workers, it is often difficult to navigate the second career job market. That's where the Seoul 50 Plus Foundation comes in—to help the roughly 3.5 million middle-aged residents prepare for that next act. The foundation offers an array of services, including training, job fairs, and job placement assistance. At the foundation's offices, I'm briefed on a new internship program, inspired by the Robert De Niro movie *The Intern*, that matches up "retired" executives with small technology start-up companies. I was a little startled that a middling Hollywood flick could drive policy in Korea, and to be fair, my hosts seemed a little sheepish about the program's origin story, but a good idea is a good idea, and the program has found fertile ground with business executives seeking to use their skills in a next-act career.

Roughly two hundred people go through the program every year. I'm introduced to the story of Kim Jun-seok, who retired at age sixty-four after a career as an executive at Korean Air and Hallym Hospital. Kim thought he had finally reached his well-earned rest, but instead he quickly became bored, disconnected as he was from the networks and work goals that had structured his life for forty years. Hearing of the internship program, he jumped at the chance to work at an early-stage new media PR firm named Ruwa Content. Kim was not dissuaded by the short-term assignment (three months), or the fact that the average age of the staff was twenty-eight, or that the CEO was young enough to be his son. He wasn't even turned off by the minimum wage pay that amounted to only six hundred thousand won (roughly $450) a month. Kim needed a new challenge, and fortunately for him, Ruwa Content was in equal need, with rampant turnover and a CEO who was struggling to manage a young but growing company. There were cultural challenges—Kim shed his ties in favor of blue jeans—but in three months, he systemized wages, created a pay-for-performance plan, and brought a new culture of professionalism to the company. At the end of three months, he re-upped, not as an intern but as the company's chief operating officer, presumably making more than minimum wage. In the end, Kim's story hardly resembles a Hollywood movie—plots are not typically built around revising HR systems—but it does reflect the effort to keep the professional class active and engaged.[37]

There are enormous changes going on in the huge office towers that dot Seoul and Busan, but at the street level, I mostly see older workers in the small shops and markets that were the foundation of the Korean economy forty years ago and still provide much of its economic culture. Early one morning, I take the subway out to Noryangjin Fish Market, the main wet market for Seoul. It's a vast hangar, several football fields in length, of fish stalls, each individually owned and family-staffed. The assortment of fish is astonishing: lobsters, clams, eels, king crabs, snow crabs, skate, giant tuna, flounder, red snapper, squid—an entire aquarium of life. You don't have to worry about the freshness of the fish here, because mostly they are still alive, at least until they are not. There is a lot of death going on here, dealt by knives and scalpels, pikes and spikes, and even culinary scissors ripping across still-beating flesh. If one of the fishmongers had pulled out a mace and started wailing away at one of the bigger fish, I would not have been surprised.

Many, maybe most, of the workers are older, and many of them are women. The woman slicing away at a still-protesting octopus is about sixty-five. Her neighbor in the next stall over is pushing seventy-five, and the woman holding up the three-foot-wide king crab for my inspection is a few years older than that. There is of course an age range in the large workforce inside Noryangjin, but the biggest group by far is women over the age of sixty-five. In the US and Europe, we associate manual labor with the strength of youth, or at least the plateau of middle age, but in Korea, I've seen older people, mostly women, occupy some of the hardest, on-your-feet jobs there are: waitress, cook, fishmonger, and plenty more. To a certain extent, it reflects the increasing physical capacities of older people, especially older women, but it also reflects irreplaceable skills honed over decades. Learning how to gut a tuna in five minutes and keep your dress spotless is not something you can do overnight.

———

As I travel back from Noryangjin to Itaewon, I pass a long series of skyscraper-lined office blocks, the towering buildings badged with the names of blue-chip Korean companies like Samsung, SK, and POSCO. It's easy for me to imagine the legions of older workers in those offices—this is Korea, after all—for the most part comfortably ensconced at their desks. They may be of the same generation as the women of Noryangjin, but the physical challenges are a world apart. I'm full of admiration for the skills and physical stamina of these older women, but the price that they pay for hard, on-your-feet labor year after year, decade after decade, can be a steep one. I've talked with hundreds of older workers over the years, and most have told me that they work because they want to, but as you descend the economic ladder, the mix of motivations changes. In Korea, a country that has traditionally relied on the family as the social safety net, many older workers now have to keep working out of necessity. There are many profound inequalities when it comes to work, and they don't end when you get older.

But work is still a respite from the loneliness of life, especially in the later years, and that is doubly true for blue-collar workers. Just as both pay and physical comfort at work are often inequitably distributed among white-collar and blue-collar workers, so is social connection, and usually in the same direction. In the United States, for example, 33 percent of college graduates report having six or more friends. That's not an encouraging figure; it has shrunk considerably over the years, but it's positively communal compared to high school graduates, where the number of people with six or more friends has collapsed to 17 percent. The number of high school graduates reporting zero friends stands at a frightening 24 percent, an 800 percent increase from twenty-five years ago and easily double the same figure for college graduates.[38] We can feel mixed emotions, I certainly do, about extending careers for blue-collar workers, but let's not buy into the airbrushed picture of retirement. For many blue-collar workers, retirement means little more than reduced circumstances and the loss of remaining social networks.

I see older blue-collar workers all over Seoul, but that's partly because I am looking for them. In relative terms, their numbers are in sharp decline, simply because there are far fewer blue-collar jobs. In the United States of 1970, blue-collar jobs accounted for 32 percent of total nonfarm employment. By 2016, their share had fallen by more than half, to 13.6 percent of total employment.[39] Korea, and virtually all economically advanced economies, has also experienced various levels of decline. With the rise in workforce automation and artificial intelligence, that percentage is almost certain to continue to shrink. The questions and opportunities around older workers will continue to be nuanced, but with the rise of assistive technology, the decline in blue-collar jobs, and the increase in physical capacity, the arc of work will continue to bend toward older workers.

There are already more than one billion people over the age of sixty alive right now, but by 2050, that number will more than double to 2.1 billion.[40] In the US, the aging of the historically large Baby Boomer generation has meant momentous changes in the number of people sixty-five and older, from 39.7 million in 2009 to about fifty-eight million today, and an expected eighty-two million by mid-century. By 2035, the number of people in the United States over the age of sixty-five will outnumber the people under eighteen for the first time in history. It's the same story in the UK. Over the last forty years, the population over sixty-five has increased by over 3.5 million, a 52 percent increase. And the increase in the older population, with the aging of the Baby Boomer generation, will only accelerate. The number of people over the age of eighty, the fastest-growing segment in the UK population, is projected to double by 2060.

I could go on, country by country, describing our new super-aged society, but the story is fundamentally the same everywhere: Rapid increases in the number of older people are fundamentally reengineering the demographic structure of our world. If it was just the supercharged growth in the number of older people, that would probably be manageable within the scope of existing economic systems, but the growth in older adults is matched by a rapid decline in births. For the last half century, birth rates around the world have plunged, from five births per woman in 1950 to just 2.3 in 2021. In the United States, the fertility rate has fallen all the way to a record low of 1.62 births per woman as of 2023, down from 3.65 in 1960. It's a stunning decline, but it is the envy of countries like Korea, Italy, and Japan, whose rates have consistently dipped below one birth per woman. Korea's birth rate is a quarter of what it was just a half century ago.

People in some quarters may celebrate the decline in birth rate, believing that our planet cannot sustain growing populations. It's not a view shared in Seoul. The skyrocketing costs of childcare and housing and the high pressures of the country's educational and work systems have driven more and more families to postpone having children or even to eschew them altogether. Countries like Japan and Korea that have highly restrictive immigration policies are left with burgeoning populations of older people and shrinking populations of younger people. If no changes are made, Korea's population will fall in half by the end of the century, with the population significantly weighted toward the older end of the spectrum.

People who work on aging and longevity issues just hate it when all of this is described as the "silver tsunami." They consider it irredeemably ageist to associate the increasing number of older people with a meteorological disaster. It's a fair point—we're constantly undermining a perfectly natural human progression with negative language—but here it's at once both ageist and accurate: The crosscurrents of greater life expectancy and plunging birth rates threaten to undermine global economies worse than any storm could. In places like Korea, it is not clear that they will have enough workers to sustain the economy or pay the costs of all those long-lived retirees. Japan, which already has the highest labor participation rate among older people, will need to substantially increase the work rates of older adults just to keep its labor force at current levels.

Perhaps extraordinary advances in productivity, maybe from AI, will allow growth even with a shrinking labor force, but from a public policy perspective, that seems like a rather speculative bet.

Even the US, which has historically benefited from high immigration rates, will still struggle to deal with the increasing number of retirees. In 1940, in the early days of Social Security, the dependency ratio, the number of active workers to retirees, was forty-two. By 1955, that had fallen all the way to 8.6 workers per retiree, and today it is under three.[41] It is estimated that in OECD countries, in order to maintain the current balance between working-age and non-working-age populations, by 2050, retirement ages would need to increase by an estimated 8.4 years.[42] The potential consequences of an increasing imbalance between workers and retirees are profound and scary, and might include everything from an overtaxed retirement system to declining growth and an inadequate labor force.

Governments around the world have struggled with this challenge for decades, but changes in retirement and pension rules have surprisingly little effect on actual retirement behavior. In the US, despite repeated increases to the date of eligibility for full Social Security benefits, the actual age of retirement for Americans has barely budged over the last six decades. In 1960, men on average retired at age sixty-six. Today, the number is sixty-five.[43]

Don't blame the men. They work in an environment that remains hostile to older workers. According to AARP, only 4 percent of employers worldwide have tried to implement human resource programs to accommodate older workers. In the US, two-thirds of older workers believe age discrimination is common in the workplace. One in five older workers have reported that they have directly experienced age discrimination, and one in four have heard negative comments about an older worker's age. Companies prize the perceived innovation and technology savvy of younger workers—as well as their lower salaries—so older workers are often the first out during periods of economic austerity, and they are at a tremendous disadvantage when trying to find new work. The reemployment rate for workers over sixty-two is only 38 percent, barely half of what it is for younger workers. And those who do find work usually do so with a substantial salary haircut, on average about 29 percent less than what they made before.[44] It's pretty awful to be an older worker in the US, and it's not much better in the UK. One in three British adults over the age of fifty report being turned down for a job because of their age, and older job seekers are, according to the Centre for Ageing Better, "less likely to be hired and, once employed, less likely to receive training."[45]

Compare that to countries like Japan where companies are an integral part of a larger movement to rethink work practices in light of population aging. Ultimately, it will take collaboration among government, workers, and companies to effect meaningful change, and at least in countries like the US and the UK, we remain far from achieving that.

———

Singapore has several advantages in the battle of the aging work-force. Older people want to keep on working—77 percent of Singaporeans over sixty say they want to stay employed—and the government has created a string of financial incentives, including cash payments to companies that develop reemployment policies or flexible work arrangements for older workers. It's part of a strategy that is one part economics and one part healthy aging. As Lim Sia

Hoe, the energetic director of the Centre for Seniors in Singapore tells me, the government knows that "so long as seniors are thinking, working, or being engaged, they stay healthy. . . . [Work gives seniors] a way to engage with friends and their work colleagues. They find satisfaction. . . . They find themselves."

Despite the incentives from the government, Singaporean companies remain reluctant to recruit older workers and create advantageous working conditions for them. Singapore trails Japan, Korea, and even the US in providing jobs for older workers, and that has left the government with lots of older employees wanting to work and not enough outlets for them—and a need to rapidly innovate.

Lim Sia Hoe introduces me to one such innovation, a new "micro jobs" program offering high-purpose work with shorter, flexible hours created by the Thye Hua Kwan Moral Charities (THK). THK runs one of the largest active aging networks in Singapore, with eighteen centers spread across the city. Traditionally, the centers have been "senior centers" focused on activities most relevant to the "old old." But with the mandate to strengthen lifelong health, the mission of THK has broadened to include supporting the "young old" and ensuring that they stay engaged, productive, and active. In January, just a few months before I visited Singapore, THK launched its micro jobs program and within weeks, more than two hundred seniors were on the payroll.

I visited THK on a Wednesday, and by Thursday I was a microjobber too, walking rounds with Shu Teng Lee, age seventy-three and a former manager of a manufacturing company. Five days a week, he delivers meals to about thirty seniors, some older than him, some younger. His daily route starts at Block 90, a lower-income housing building adjacent to the local THK center. Shu then hops on his bike to deliver the second half of the meals to a more distant housing block. His work solves a last-mile problem for the Meals on Wheels program, allowing meals to be dropped off at a central location and farming out the delivery to seniors from other seniors.

Shu sees his work as a civic duty—this is organized by a "moral charity," after all—to help others who do not share his good health. Helping others is the first thing he mentions among reasons for participating in the program, but he is keenly aware of the link between activity and health: "I can't sit around at home. It would kill me." He gets paid for the work. The amount matters less to him—it comes out to about twenty Singaporean dollars a day—but the pay confirms this as a serious obligation, one that he can't wave away if he doesn't feel like doing it. It's a job, and the rituals and rules of work apply.

Together, we carry fourteen sets of meals up to Block 90. Like 80 percent of the housing in Singapore, it's public housing owned by the Singapore Housing and Development Board (HDB). The HDB is one of the largest apartment owners in the world, and it updates its buildings with remarkable efficiency. It's called the Great Construction. Once a building hits fifty years, all residents are rotated out to new homes, pulling along all the adjoining eateries, beauty salons, and other shops that make a neighborhood a neighborhood. The old building comes down, to be replaced with a brand-new apartment complex. Many of the new buildings are architectural wonders worthy of entry in global design competitions. That's not Block 90. Judging from the flickering lights and weathered cinderblocks, Block 90 must be nearing its expiration date. Bicycles cram the corridors, and cooking smells tiptoe out of the apartments as we move down the dim hallways. Block 90, unlike newer facilities, lacks air-conditioning, so many doors are open to catch whatever small cross breeze there may be on this hot, sticky day. It's all in vain, as the air is completely still inside the building, and my shirt soaks through, not for the first time that day.

Shu knocks on doors and double-checks his list to ensure that the meals go to the right people. It's a daily routine, though all the residents are rather startled to find not only Shu but me, my microphones, and my two young handlers from the National University. Shu greets the "auntie" or the "uncle" within, inquiring after their health and well-being. It's part of the job, as Shu has responsibility not just for delivering the meals, but also for keeping tabs on socially isolated seniors, spotting any problems, and connecting them with services as the case may require.

We finish our rounds. It's only been thirty minutes, though the oppressive heat makes it feel much longer. Shu loads up his bicycle for the next set of deliveries, and he expresses gratitude that he can still work. "I'm so fortunate that I can help. A few of them are younger than me, but they are already in wheelchairs. . . . So I feel that, really, I'm very grateful that I'm so good. So that's why I like to help." I wish Shu continued good health and good luck. He laughs and invites me back to join him again, in twenty years, in 2044. I may not make it, but I wouldn't bet against Shu still being at it in his nineties.

Three Tips for Healthy Aging

What does this mean for Table 23?

Keep working. The work revolution is here, or at least it's headed in that direction in many parts of the world. Older people increasingly want to work—and the numbers of older people with functional limitations and those who need help with the activities of daily living are declining.[46] Even in the United States, workers over the age of seventy-five are the fastest-growing part of the workforce, more than quadrupling in size since 1964. Some 9 percent of adults aged seventy-five and older are employed, about twice the share who were working as recently as 1987.[47] Call it whatever you want—not retiring, unretirement, or working in retirement—it is already a trend and will reshape our notions of work and the workforce.

For Table 23, the future begins with recognizing that the conventions around retirement—that we should all retire by age sixty-five—are to a certain extent arbitrary in the first place and likely to continue to erode in the face of changing demographics and capabilities. We should perceive work as instrumental not just to our financial planning, but also to our health planning. It's not for everyone—even in Japan and Korea there are plenty of people living in traditional retirement—but careful planning for the years past sixty requires thinking about work as an option, and how it can help fill our needs for social connection, meaning, and mobility.

Be present. Remote working tripled in response to COVID-19, and it hasn't returned to anywhere near pre-pandemic levels despite the best efforts of CEOs, HR teams, and now the president.[48] There are many advantages to remote work: I work at home myself, and it is particularly attractive to caregivers, the disabled, and many older adults. Without a doubt, the flexibility that remote technology offers will be an ingredient of the workplace of the future. But what technology gives with one hand, it takes with the other. Remote work is increasingly part of our isolated, lonely lives, and it is particularly hard on older workers. According to Gallup, a full 25 percent of remote workers already admit to loneliness, and putting a wall of technology between coworkers is not helping. Work is one of the few sources of social connection that has not declined in modern American society, but even that has changed in the post-pandemic world. Some twenty-two million American workers are now fully remote, and tens of millions more work in a hybrid format, to the detriment of social cohesion. The share of US workers who say they know coworkers on a personal level has fallen from 80 percent in 2019 to 67 percent in 2024.[49] In January 2020, 47 percent of American workers believed someone at work cared about them. Now it's just 38 percent. The emptying of American offices has even engendered loneliness in those left behind, as some 19 percent of on-site workers report being lonely for "a lot" of the day.

We as humans are a deeply tactile species: Our sense of well-being, our humanity really, is tied to face-to-face contact. A 2024 study of nearly thirteen thousand people found that having face-to-face contact with friends at least once a week was a strong predictor of better physical and mental health. I love the immediacy of texting, but it's the fast food of human connection: briefly satisfying, but terrible for you in the long run. The same 2024 study showed that calling or texting just don't bring the same benefits as in-person contact. There are many factors, some unrelated to work geography, that impact loneliness at work, and simply bringing people back to the office won't in and of itself change our slide downward.[50] But it is the place to start. My advice to Table 23 is to make sure that there is a face-to-face component in any work they may choose to do.[51]

Be flexible with work. Everyone has a different measure of what constitutes a good job. But as you get older, requirements change. Prioritize flexible, interactive work at companies that care about older workers. Look for companies, including those that have taken the AARP Employer Pledge in the US, the Age-Friendly Employer Pledge in the UK, or the Inter-Company Commitment on Workers over Fifty in France, for example, that evidence interest in older workers, which can be shown by their support for flex work, part-time work, job sharing, intergenerational mentorships, and the like.[52] The evaluation of what constitutes "good work" for older workers should be concentrated on the social value that it provides, the purpose it brings to workers, and the social connections that it affords to coworkers and to customers. Japan has one of the most competitive work environments in the world, but older workers are increasingly valuing jobs that are physically active and socially engaged. We're not that different in the United States. According to the Harris Poll, 79 percent of hiring managers say that there are more older workers applying for entry-level jobs than just three years ago. I don't discount the economic element of the story and the difficulties that older workers have in finding jobs commensurate with their skills, but it also reflects a new trend where older workers value flexibility, learning new skills, and interacting with other people more than traditional incentives related to prestige.[53] For most older people, staying active and engaged is the single most important thing you can do for your health—and work is the most readily available avenue.

Chapter 3

All Mixed Up

L UZ GRASPS MY forearm—it's a firm grip, certainly for an eighty-eight-year-old—and startles me by breaking into song. I don't recognize it, which is not terribly surprising since my personal catalogue of songs starts around 1976 and ends not too many years later. And it's in Spanish, which also makes sense, since we are in Ourense, just north of the border with Portugal. Luz has a strong voice, though not a particularly good one, but that doesn't stop her from singing with wonderful enjoyment and gusto. She finishes the song, and before I can applaud, she launches on to the next.

It's a rather swift turn because moments before, Luz had introduced herself to me with a melancholy shrug, claiming that she was tired—not of the moment, but of life. It's always a difficult thing to hear, though I've heard it on more than one occasion from the very old, an admission that death would be a release from the physical pain and limitations of late life and a welcome reunion with people who have gone before. But it turns out, Luz is a bit of a performer, offering up the tired old lady character before she swiftly transforms into the ancient diva, singing songs for all who care to hear.

It's a good act, and it instantly attracts a tiny group of admirers: tiny in the sense that it numbers only two or three people, but also tiny in the sense that the other listeners, who grab at her feet much as she had latched onto my arm, are themselves only two or three years old. Luz gently, lovingly, shoos them away, and she confesses to me that while late life wears on her from time to time, these children, all eighty of them spread across the yard and school rooms, are "my life." Luz has spent much of her life working on farms, but now approaching the end of her ninth decade, she has found renewed purpose with these children—helping them get dressed as they go out to play, frolicking with them in the playground, and even teaching them the tricks of the trade in the little garden that occupies much of the courtyard dividing the senior center and the preschool.

The Ourense Intergenerational Center houses a senior center with about forty regular attendees, ages fifty to almost 100, and eighty children, ages zero to three. It is a lovely place: wide, generous hallways; clean lines; soft, pleasant lighting that stands in stark contrast to the harsh institutional feel of many congregate care facilities for the elderly. There are big bay windows on the senior center side, affording the elders a view of the children playing in the courtyard. If you want to venture out, even in rainy weather, there is a covered veranda where the oldsters can sit and watch. But more often than not, even on the rainy Tuesday when I visit, they walk across like Luz to join the children in the preschool area, on the playground, or in the garden. The center is run by the Provincial Government of Galicia, but it was originally funded by the

Amancio Ortega Foundation, the philanthropic arm of the owner of the clothing company Zara and a man widely reported to be the richest person in Spain.[1] The financial kicker provided by Ortega has allowed the center to add a few extras, like an exercise and rehab center for the seniors and a kitchen where the old and the young can explore food and cooking together. The Ourense Intergenerational Center is a statement, made possible by Ortega, about the profound relationship between the young and the old. And in a world drifting apart, it's a testament to the critical need to bring them together and provide guidance, support, and love for the young, as well as purpose, reciprocal love, and good health for the oldest among us.

———

There is significant evidence from evolutionary anthropology and developmental psychology that the old and the young are built for each other. Older people, as they move into the later phases of life, are driven by a deep desire to nurture the next generation. The young in turn need to be nurtured. It's a fit that goes back to the beginning of human history, what Marc Freedman, the founder of the intergenerational advocacy organization CoGenerate and the author of a number of very good books on the topic, has described as the "jigsaw puzzle" of human development.[2]

Older people have an instinct for meaningful relationships, driven in part by a growing sense of mortality, that there are fewer days ahead than behind. Call it the headstone imperative, that our contributions to life are not through our résumés but through the people we invest in and the memories we leave behind. We, they—at sixty-one, I'm not sure of the right pronoun anymore—have a deeply honed instinct to connect in ways that "flow down the generational chain," and older people have skills—patience, wisdom, insights, emotional regulation—that are evolutionarily honed to support the youngest among us. But modern society has done all that it can to disrupt the critical links between young and old: The shrinking of family size, the great urbanization that has put physical distance between generations, and generational segregation reflected in seniors-only communities have all disrupted evolutionary design. The Ourense Intergenerational Center is a statement that what society has torn asunder, it can bring back together—and when it does, good things will follow for all generations.

For older generations, the good things include better health outcomes, decreased mortality, and better quality of life. As we know, strong, close personal relationships are the key to happiness and vitality, and that translates directly into who lives longer and more healthfully. But some relationships are better than others. Adults with strong intergenerational relationships are *three times* as likely to be happy as those without. If you're looking for a hidden key to your health, strong and proximate intergenerational relationships would be a good place to start your search.

It's taken me a long time to grasp why there should be a strong correlation between personal health and what Erik Erikson, the great child psychoanalyst and expert on psychosocial development, has labeled "generativity," the role that each generation plays in molding and guiding the next. Generativity takes many forms, including procreating and taking parenting responsibility for the family unit, but as we get older, it ripens into a broader concern for the next generation, to support the village as it moves forward beyond our own years. Generativity, research has shown, plays a crucial role in the development of successful communities and resilient individuals—the single best predictive factor of success for an at-risk youth is the existence of a caring adult outside the immediate family such as a mentor, teacher, or other adult who takes them under their wing. Evolution rewards adults, especially older adults, who support younger generations; the critical role that grandmothers play in family success is one of the biological explanations for why women live longer than men. Generativity provides meaning and purpose to life, which in turn leads to lower inflammation, higher immunities, and better mental health. There is a critical evolutionary transaction here: Older people who invest in younger generations are rewarded with better health.[3]

You can see it over and over again in health research. Studies from Spain, China, Portugal, the UK, and Canada, among many other countries, have found positive impacts on health, well-being, and cognitive abilities.[4] In 2019, a team of researchers from Hong Kong studied the role of intergenerational relationships among older Chinese in the United States.[5] This is a particularly instructive population to study because Chinese immigrants to the US have moved from a society that emphasizes respect for elders and has a high percentage of multigenerational households to one that has neither. While this is a much-studied population by anthropologists, it was the first study of Chinese immigrants that directly dove into the impact of multigenerational relationships on health—and found that the sense of closeness with children and grandchildren was a critical determinant of health.

Close intergenerational connections have a mediative effect on happiness, emotional stability, and meaning and purpose, all of which contribute significantly to better health. In Latino communities in the US, the positive health effects of strong intergenerational relationships are a contributor to what is known as the "Hispanic Paradox," the longer life expectancy of Latinos in the US compared to Whites and other demographic groups despite comparatively low income and other socioeconomic disadvantages.[6] It is what I saw in Presidio, Texas, and other communities striped across the southern tier of the US.

The strength of intergenerational ties in many immigrant communities in the United States is a strong contributor to health and stability amid an often-charged political and social atmosphere, which makes it even more of a pity that those bonds tend to loosen in second- and third-generation families as immigrants become acculturated to "American" practices.[7] The Hispanic Paradox—and better health and life expectancy—tends to weaken in successive generations as younger people become divorced from traditional norms. Americans might be inclined to think of it as part of the natural order for generations to spread apart only to reconvene to spar over the Thanksgiving table, but a growing body of evidence suggests that strong intergenerational relationships in fact have been a key to human development itself all along—and a key to successful and healthy aging.

———

Research published in 2013 by demographer Richelle Winkler shows that in the US, age segregation is often as ingrained as racial segregation. Using census data from 1990 to 2010, Winkler found that in some parts of the country, old (age sixty and over) and young (age twenty to thirty-four) are roughly as segregated as Latinos and Whites, a sobering finding in a country where most Latinos live in neighborhoods that are less than one-third White[8] and the average Latino elementary school student typically attends a school with only 30 percent White attendance.[9] And it is a growing trend: Between the 1990s and 2010, the number of neighborhoods experiencing age segregation grew by about a third.[10] We consider de facto racial segregation a major societal problem, but age segregation is deemed a feature rather than a bug, the natural way of living. The US has been described as the "most age segregated society that's ever been," but in most quarters that is greeted with a collective shrug.[11] We celebrate the nuclear family and, though the norm was challenged during the COVID-19 pandemic, we still largely expect children to "leave the nest" at the earliest possible opportunity.

And social approbation follows if you don't. Whenever I think about American culture and the multigenerational family, my mind often takes me to the decidedly mainstream, but also surprisingly weird, 2006 rom-com *Failure to Launch*. In the movie, Matthew McConaughey plays Tripp, a thirty-five-year-old bachelor content to live with his parents and take full advantage of their seemingly bottomless hospitality. His parents, however, are less satisfied with this arrangement, but their hints to Tripp to move on are routinely ignored or rebuffed. Desperate, they hire Paula, played by Sarah Jessica Parker, who has an improbable expertise in convincing grown men to move out of their parents' house. Paula's ploy is to "befriend" these men, building up their confidence so that they can finally screw up the courage to leave the safety of the family nest. No plot holes or ethical problems there, but fortunately for Paramount Pictures, the movie tapped into a broader cultural concern of the time that young people were too pampered and were slowly undermining American values of individualism and self-reliance. That plus the winsome combination of McConaughey and Parker turned the film into a domestic box office success.

———

You never want to take too much away from Hollywood's imagining of American values, but in *Failure to Launch* there was an uncomfortable kernel of truth in an otherwise contrived plot. The economic imperatives of industrialization and urbanization of the twentieth century pulled families and generations apart, and as often happens, social values were developed to dress up economic rules. Few people in America realize that the highly age-segregated nature of work, friendships, and living arrangements is a recent creation of modern society. Well into the nineteenth century, the vast majority of Americans lived in multigenerational housing, often on the farm. People lived, labored, and socialized in intergenerational units. But the great wave of urbanization of the early twentieth century and the ascendency of the nuclear family changed not only how we live, but who we interact with on a regular basis.

Failure to Launch mostly focused on people in midlife—the actors who played Tripp's parents were in their fifties—but the generational divide is most acute, and most felt, when it comes to later life. Over time, many older Americans have been persuaded to believe that a happy retirement means leaving community and a lifetime of relationships to move to a place inhabited only by other older people. It reflects the growing challenge in the United States that we really don't know what to do with all these old people.

It's an issue that is again of recent vintage. In an America deeply enthralled with a national image of youth and vigor, the whole concept of retirement and old age has been viewed as a bit of an embarrassing problem. In the early twentieth century, the number of senior citizens in the United States was only about three million, and solutions were mostly local. But by the middle of the century, the number of adults over the age of sixty-five had ballooned to twelve million—and the challenge of what to do with all these old people could no longer be ignored.

Into that void came "Big Ben" Schleifer, who in 1955 launched Youngtown, the first fifty-five and older community in the country. Schleifer had moved to Phoenix from Rochester, New York, six years earlier in hopes that the dry air would cure his asthma, but his interest in senior living had been roused on trips back to Rochester where he saw elderly friends confined to nursing homes, mired in lonely, isolated conditions. Big Ben was an idealist, a communitarian who wanted to create a new town that would allow older people of modest means to find a place of shared interests, acceptance, and common purpose, a condition mostly reserved for the young in an America captivated with the notion of youthful vigor and power. "Live Here and Be Forever Young" was the motto and aspirational goal of Youngtown. Schleifer built 125 homes in the first year and sold just eighty-four, a rather meager start, but Youngtown captured a piece of the national consciousness, if not the real estate market, when it was featured in Dave Garroway's national TV show *Wide, Wide World*.

Big Ben was an idea man, but he proved not to be the right person to turn a grand vision into a successful business. Youngtown still exists, but it never grew substantially beyond the early years and lost its legal designation as an age-restricted community in 1998. The task of turning Big Ben's vision into a fundamental reimagination of how we live instead fell to the legendary real estate developer Del Webb.[12]

Webb was a sprawling and controversial figure, at the time the owner of the New York Yankees. He made his considerable fortune building some of the largest Japanese American internment camps in World War II and later helping the mobster Bugsy Siegel develop the Flamingo Hotel in Las Vegas. After he saw the Youngtown story reported by Garroway, he became seized by the idea of persuading older Americans to abandon their hometowns in favor of retirement in the burning southwestern desert. It was a bold idea but was viewed skeptically by many within the Del Webb Development Company. To prove out the concept, Webb dispatched Tom Breen, one of his chief lieutenants, to Clearwater, Florida, to assess the status of the American retiree. Breen's method of real estate due diligence was unusual—he sat on park benches and chatted up passing retirees—but he returned with a positive report on the idea. Webb sprang into action, sinking millions of dollars into building the first modern retirement community, complete with golf courses and pools and many of the amenities we recognize as commonplace today. In 1959 he christened Sun City, immediately adjacent to Youngtown. Unlike Youngtown it was a runaway success. Cars lined the streets just to drive by the model homes, and 237 units were sold on the first weekend. Webb sold over two thousand homes in that first year and launched a boom in senior housing.

The success of Sun City spawned endless imitators, and today there are more than sixteen thousand senior living communities in the United States. They range from single-building operations to the oft-ridiculed yet astonishingly successful community of The Villages in central Florida, which was the fastest-growing metropolitan area in the entire United States during the last decade. As the country has aged, senior living communities have gotten both bigger, as with The Villages, and more niche, like communities dedicated to everything from Zen philosophy to the recently deceased singer Jimmy Buffet and his legion of still-loyal Parrot Heads.[13] After seventy years, the senior living business has both embraced a certain kind of diversity and maintained a singular commitment to walling off older people from the rest of the world.

It's fashionable in some quarters, my quarters to be specific, to ridicule places like The Villages for its libertine atmosphere (almost certainly an urban myth) and its conservative politics (true, but consistent with the rest of rural Florida), but people keep coming. The active aging market segment, as it is called, is expected to reach about $800 billion by 2030, and it's not difficult to see why. Two years ago, a few days before Christmas, with the long-suffering Nate in tow, I visited The Villages. If nothing else, The Villages are an extraordinary business success story. The community started just thirty years ago as a few dozen mobile homes tucked into a corner of a poor central Florida county, but today it sprawls eighteen miles across three counties, seventy-five thousand homes, 150,000 residents, and a plan to double that in the next decade.

And truth be told, The Villages does a lot right. In an era marked by increasing loneliness, especially among older adults, The Villages makes it hard to be alone. There are 127 recreational centers in The Villages, and each has some two dozen planned activities per day. On the day we were there, we witnessed water volleyball, bridge, pottery, and pickleball but somehow missed out on tap dancing, team shuffleboard, a World War II book club meeting, and cardio drumming. I had never heard of cardio drumming before my visit, but there are ten affinity groups dedicated to just that subject, plus thirteen genealogical groups, sixteen mah-jongg clubs, and sixty-four music groups, including a drumming group for those who like drums but are not interested in the cardio part of it. There are seven movie clubs, seven remote-controlled boat clubs, seven pinochle clubs, seven political clubs (three liberal, three conservative, and one ambiguously called We the People), and since seven seems to be the answer to the question of how many clubs there are in The Villages on every conceivable subject, seven trivia clubs. And if I get stuck trying to figure out how to end this paragraph, I can seek support from one of the thirteen writer's clubs.

Don't get me wrong. It's still easy to troll The Villages. It's almost exclusively white in a state that is verging on majority-minority, and its attempts to conjure other places and times are painfully inauthentic. Brownwood Paddock Square recalls a nineteenth-century Florida cattle town just as much as *Hogan's Heroes* evoked a real German POW camp. And the secretive family concern that runs The Villages works very hard to isolate it from the surrounding communities. Drive through The Villages, and you will see mile after mile of tidy middle-class homes and closely cropped lawns. Walk across any street that marks the outer boundaries of The Villages, and you will discover a more common look of rural Florida: dilapidated shotgun shacks, busted-out cars, and unrelenting poverty—but I don't get the sense that anyone ever bothers to cross that street.

People who live in The Villages might cross the street to greet a child, but there aren't many. Children can visit, but they can't live there, and I didn't see any during my visit. Maggie Kuhn, the founder of the Gray Panthers, once dismissed age-restricted communities as "glorified playpens," but that doesn't feel quite right to me. These places wouldn't be so successful if they didn't fill a need in people's lives, to be where they are valued, where they are central to the life of the neighborhood rather than shunted aside as too often happens in American communities. But they are incomplete. I'd rather think of them, echoing Freedman's description, as jigsaw puzzles missing some of the critical pieces; it might be fun for a while, but in the end, it will leave you unsatisfied and more than a bit frustrated.[14]

It's not all in one direction, of course. Indeed, starting even before the COVID-19 pandemic, there has been a substantial increase in intergenerational living arrangements in the United States.[15] This increase has been driven at least in significant part by the rapid rise in housing costs. Social expectations around the age when younger people should appropriately leave the nest have begun to change in the wake of economic imperatives. And there is even a modest movement to create "shared sites" that intentionally bring the generations together. Researchers at Ohio State University and the advocacy group Generations United have catalogued some 105 places in the United States that pair young and old together in the same location.[16] It's mostly cohousing developments like Bridge Meadows in Oregon, with lots of interesting variations on the model: Nesterly is a technology platform that helps older homeowners sublet rooms to students, and Mirabella is a retirement housing complex that is integrated into the campus and curriculum of Arizona State University. These are remarkable projects led by people of unusual vision and commitment, but on the "how we live" map of the United States, they amount to barely a pinprick. And that's because we don't associate intergenerational relationships with better health, or with much of anything. If you asked

Americans for a list of the strategies for healthy aging, intergenerational relationships would not register at all.

Places like The Villages are not the root cause of generational isolation in the US, but they certainly reflect it. And that's also probably why active aging communities have not found similar purchases in other countries, especially the ones profiled here. It is true that a string of retirement communities has sprung up in Spain, with age-restricted facilities dotting the Costa del Sol, the Costa de la Cruz, and the Balearic Islands. But most of those communities cater largely to foreigners seeking the sun, the advantageous cost structure of Spain, and ways of living in retirement that are familiar to them. They are far less successful with older Spaniards, who continue to prefer the social connection, intergenerational support, and sense of purpose provided by integrating into a multigenerational society, not separating from it.

———

It's very different in Singapore too. When the Ministry of Health adopted its first Action Plan for Successful Ageing in 2015, it laid out some seventy major programs to support the goal of helping older Singaporeans be healthier, more productive, and more socially connected. Very few of the programs specifically focused on intergenerational relationships or even mentioned them. They didn't need to, because the goal of fostering and supporting a generationally integrated society was threaded throughout the effort. In Singapore, generational comity forms the baseline for furthering healthy aging, and it reflects a cultural consensus that all generations are better off when they are brought together in a meaningful way.

The Kampung Admiralty Hawker Centre, even at eleven in the morning, is cooking. Pots clang, cashiers call out orders, and hundreds of customers chat away in what is essentially a sweaty outdoor food court. I take my tray of fish ball soup to a side table where I can watch the scene. My fish balls are a little disappointing—nicely chewy, but bland and not nearly as memorable as the name suggests. But the Hawker Centre doesn't disappoint. There is an energy in the room that speaks to the role of Kampung Admiralty as a community crossroads, where people from all over can come together, bump into one another, and connect. Kampung means "village," and Kampung Admiralty, a mix of housing, restaurants, shopping, and services, has been designed to be the center of this neighborhood in central Singapore.

Nothing too surprising there, except for the fact that Kampung Admiralty is a retirement village with its 100-plus units reserved for people fifty-five and older. In our age-stratified society, it's unusual to think of a retirement village as an attraction point—the object is often to keep the young people out—but Kampung Admiralty is entirely different. It sits on top of the Admiralty metro step, making it the necessary first stop for anyone passing through, as tens of thousands do each day. The restaurants of the Hawker Centre and the ground floor below draw a mixed-age crowd. As I sit there pushing my fish balls around my bowl, I can see that the largest group is older residents, but the crowd is substantially leavened by dozens of school-age children and people in midlife. Even built and occupied as a retirement village, Kampung Admiralty has become the meeting place for the community and an intergenerational hub. It reflects the views of its designers, and really the consensus view of

Singaporeans, that integrating the generations is a key public health strategy in the struggle for longer and healthier life.

You can find it easily enough if you know what you are looking for in the shops and food stalls on the ground floors, but you can't miss it when you travel to the seventh floor, which is the province of the youngest and the oldest in the community. It is a typical Singapore design ethic now to match up young and old as a means of creating purpose and meaning for the elderly and support for the young. On one side of the elevator bank, people, mostly in their eighties and nineties I would guess, are lunching at the senior day care center, while on the other side, thirty small children, clad in matching bright orange shirts and white shorts, are similarly sitting down to their lunch. The furnishings are quite different, mostly wheelchairs on one side and the tiniest of tables on the other, but there is a metaphorical tether between the rooms. The two groups meet throughout the day, sometimes in intentional joint activities and sometimes in accidental meetings that are fostered by design.

Bringing the generations together is a bit of a mania in Singapore. In the US, there is a constituency for intergenerational activities, including groups like Generations United and CoGenerate. They do important, meaningful work, but they are tiny in the grand scheme of things, and you will never randomly bump into someone who thinks of intergenerational connection as a core public health or personal health strategy. But you will in Singapore. From the seventh floor at Kampung Admiralty, I take the elevator up to the rooftop gardens. Singapore planners use rooftop gardens to save energy and water, but also to bring people out of their apartments into community. The gardens at Kampung Admiralty are a point of pride, sprinkled with lush green trees and neatly arrayed vegetable plots. It's an oasis in the city but today in the broiling midday heat, it's not a very inviting one. The sun bakes down on the roof, roasting anyone foolish enough to test its limits. For a while I'm the only fool, but ten minutes after I arrive, the elevator doors open, and a middle-aged man walks out. We're the only ones on the roof, so we end up in conversation, as people on hot, steamy roofs tend to do. He introduces himself as Kenneth—we high-five over our shared name—and he tells me he is a health care worker taking a recertification course at a classroom in Kampung Admiralty. Maybe it's his profession, or maybe it's just Singapore, but he volunteers that he is a longevity enthusiast and completely unprompted starts telling me the importance of keeping the generations together. I'm not particularly surprised that someone in Singapore would have healthy aging on their minds—it's practically a national obsession—but I'm floored that a stranger would randomly start extolling the virtues of generativity. He also tells me to eat watermelon to keep cool, but that doesn't fit the story quite as well.

Kampung Admiralty wasn't the only roof deck I hit in Singapore. Just days later, I was standing on floor forty-seven atop Skyville @ Dawson, a public housing development in the Queenstown neighborhood. From there, I had a panoramic view stretching from the port all the way to Malaysia. Ever since I had arrived in Singapore a few days before, I had conceived of the country as one large construction site, as the city races to build one enormous apartment block after another to house the growing population. But as I stood on the roof, I could see that my ground-level impression was dead wrong. Singapore from the air is a sea of green: large parks monopolizing significant swaths of the city and bright green tendrils snaking through what from the ground seem like the densest urban jungles.

John Wong, my guide that afternoon through Queenstown, tells me that the plan for Singapore, laid out by its first prime minister, Lee Kuan Yew, was to build "a city within a garden," and they have done that with the usual Singaporean combination of vision and ruthless legalism. If the tree has a "girth of more than one metre" (basically a tree you can't put your arms around),[17] it is illegal to cut it down without the prior permission of the government, even if the tree is in your own backyard. I don't know what the penalties are for breaking that particular law, but my guess is that few bother to find out.

Singapore has brought that same enthusiasm for big ideas to the challenges of an aging population. Wong is squiring me around what is now called the Health District at Queenstown, a new urban laboratory for maximizing healthy longevity. To the American ear, the phrase "health district" typically means "unhealthy district," a place with a large concentration of hospitals, doctors, and medical services to take care of the sick. In Singapore, it means what it says: a place where the population can stay healthy and vital, and efforts are focused on keeping people that way. For Wong, who oversees the project, that means helping the 100,000 residents of Queenstown stay socially connected, purposeful, and intergenerationally engaged.[18]

Queenstown holds a central place in the story of Singapore's reinvention. As we drive around the district, Wong narrates the Queenstown he remembers from his youth: "A lot of wooden shacks, people drinking well water and pipe water that wasn't very hygienic, a lot of graveyards." It was a neighborhood emblematic of how Singapore used to be. But when the Housing and Development Board was let loose to create the new Singapore, it started in Queenstown. Today, virtually all of Queenstown that Wong knew is long gone, replaced by long rows of apartment buildings, a modern and efficient transportation system, and a series of architecturally arresting office buildings holding the headquarters of companies like Grab and Razer. Wong makes a point of swinging by the one building that he remembers fondly from his childhood, a branch of the public library, and even that is scheduled to be demolished and rebuilt into a much larger facility in the next few years. Sentimentality does not play much of a role in the ongoing transformation of Queenstown and Singapore.

Queenstown has been through a lot of reinvention in the years since independence, and so has Wong. He is a descendant of the great Chinese diaspora of the 1800s, and his family sought financial and personal security everywhere from Indonesia to Scotland before putting down permanent roots in Singapore in the middle of the last century. But even in Singapore, a majority Chinese enclave, the family faced challenges and deep-seated discrimination. Wong's grandfather, raised and educated in Scotland, had held senior medical positions there, but was unable to secure an attending position at any hospital in Singapore because they were solely reserved for Whites and the other appropriately hued offspring of the British Empire. He ended up serving the Chinese community, which seemed less bothered by his ancestry.

That didn't stop Wong from following in his grandfather's footsteps. After graduating from medical school at the National University of Singapore, Wong realized that the teaching hospitals in Singapore could not give him the well-rounded medical training he craved. With the help of his girlfriend (now wife), he wrote letters to a wide range of American hospitals and schools requesting the opportunity to apply for a residency program. He received zero responses. Unwilling to give up on his plan, he traveled to the US, starting in San Francisco and working his way east. Unable to secure appointments by mail or phone, Wong would still show up seeking an impromptu interview, but wherever he went the doctor in charge of the residency program refused to see him. Finally, having reached the East Coast and down to his last stop at Cornell University Medical College (now Weill Cornell) in New York City, Wong got in the door. He knew this was his last chance and announced to his interviewer that he was willing to work for free and had an open return ticket to Singapore, which he would use immediately if the hospital decided at any time and for any reason that they didn't need him anymore. Told to return the next day, he was presented with a contract laying out these specific terms, even though such an arrangement likely violated a shocking number of state and federal labor rules.

Signing the contract, Wong worked for free for the first year of his residency, and perhaps that would have gone on forever— they had a contract, after all. But it was seen as a manifest injustice by Wong's fellow residents, and when eighty of them threatened to walk out unless Wong was put on payroll, Cornell backed down. And perhaps they would have eventually gotten to the same place, because how would it have looked to not be paying your chief resident, which Wong became a few years later.

Returning to Singapore, Wong commenced a distinguished medical career, one that would see him named to the US National Academy of Medicine and eventually tapped to run the National University Health System (NUHS), one of the largest health care and hospital systems in the country. But as his tenure at NUHS wound down, Wong began to contemplate his next act rather than focus on the retirement he was entitled to. And perhaps appropriate for someone contemplating the later stages of life, he began to think about how the care system could be reoriented to focus on keeping people healthy, vital, and productive for longer rather than just treating them when their bodies fail. Out of this idea and a set of extensive consultations came the Health District at Queenstown, a testbed for how to keep residents active, connected, and engaged with all generations. With funding and support from a consortium that included the National University of Singapore (NUS) and the Housing and Development Board, Wong chose Queenstown for the health district not just for its historical iconography, but also its excellence in being average—the population of Queenstown closely tracks the rest of Singapore in terms of key measures such as age, income, and education.

My effort to understand generativity in Queenstown starts outside the township, at the apartment showroom of the Housing and Development Board. Just as at The Villages, how and where we live has an often-defining impact on our social connections, including with other generations. At the HDB, the goal is unmistakably pro-generational integration. That begins with the design of buildings and apartments. The HDB designs buildings with small units and generous common spaces, the better to incentivize social connections. And consistent with the city's health-building strategies, newer buildings all come with exercise courses for older adults that adjoin and thread through children's playgrounds to bring the generations together. Even the idea of buildings developed for seniors has fallen by the wayside in favor of generational integration. When I tell Wong about my visit to Kampung Admiralty and my admiration for making a senior living complex the neighborhood hub, he acknowledges the innovations of Kampung Admiralty as a first successful foray into designing public housing for older residents, but then he tells me that the next generation of housing will be different, and less segregated by age. The goal in Queenstown, and in all of Singapore now, is to design all buildings to be intergenerational: to be equally adept at serving young people, families, and older people. Housing design plays a major role in building this socially connected and intergenerational community.

At the showroom, I shed my shoes as the rules require and wander through the model apartments. I'm particularly interested in the "flexi-flats," apartments designed to help seniors age in place. They are small by American standards, but they come with key universal design elements that are attractive to seniors: Thresholds have been smoothed down to reduce trip hazards, and table heights are raised to accommodate wheelchairs. Bathrooms are wide and designed to accommodate pull bars and other accessibility features that become necessary as residents age. And in a nod to the country's focus on intergenerational activities, the HDB also offers a model colloquially called the "3Gen Flat." These units are larger, designed for greater privacy, and are reserved for multigenerational families, typically including parents, grandparents, and children all living together.

Even in family-oriented Singapore, multigenerational living is under some pressure: The number of single people under thirty-five living on their own rose by about 60 percent between 1990 and 2020. Singapore has not been exempt from the global trends—declining birth rates and smaller family size, children moving to other cities (or other countries in Singapore's case), and the cultural prominence of the nuclear family—but comparatively speaking, in

Singapore it's more of a trickle than a trend. Part of that is cultural but it also reflects the avowed policy of the central government to keep families together. The HDB supports that policy in some rather extraordinarily ham-handed ways: Unmarried people are ineligible to get an HDB apartment until age thirty-five, functionally forcing families to stay together except for the relatively small number who can afford to rent on the private market. It's a tough rule that works in the Singapore environment but probably few other places. One reason it works in Singapore is because of the tremendous control the government exercises over the housing market, but even given that, it probably wouldn't survive as a rule if it didn't reflect widespread support for the cultural norm that families should stay together. It's a concept that would come as a rather rude surprise to Kathy Bates and Terry Bradshaw, who play McConaughey's parents in *Failure to Launch*.

There are also affirmative incentives to keep families close to one another. Some rules support the notion that kids will eventually leave the nest, but that it is best if they don't go too far. Lydia Cheung, one of my guides in Singapore, lives in an apartment with her husband and young son, one floor above her in-laws. Even though apartments are largely allocated by lottery, it's not just good fortune that they ended up so close. The HDB gives preference when multigenerational families want to stay nearby. There are also tax incentives available for children who are willing to move back within one kilometer of their parents. This may seem uncomfortably close, but for Singapore and Queenstown, it is all part of supporting an intergenerational community.

Urban design and policy play an oversized role in Singapore's efforts to support generativity, but the effort is not unique to

Singapore. Just weeks after my visit to Queenstown, I am standing smack in the middle of a street in Poblenou (New Town) in the heart of Barcelona, a bubbling city of 1.7 million people and the capital of Catalonia in Spain. If it had been seven years earlier, I almost certainly would have been dodging an angry mob of cars, trucks, and buses: Barcelona has among the highest density of cars in Europe, with traffic twice that of Madrid and five times that of Berlin and Amsterdam.[19]

But today, I casually stroll down the middle of the boulevard without concern for my safety. I'm not alone. Children play in the streets, kicking a soccer ball without fear of losing it to traffic, old people sit on the benches that line the walkways that were once roads, and office workers hold meetings on the picnic tables that dot the neighborhood, invading the streets that were once the hunting grounds of automobiles. Some of the streets are even home to modern sculptures, as the neighboring art museum has turned pieces from its collection into public art. My companion on this walk, Elisa, stills our conversation, and we listen silently to the sounds of the city, people talking, kids playing, even birds chirping, sounds that would have been drowned out just a few years ago by revving engines and angry horns.

Poblenou is a superblock, a small section of Barcelona where cars are banned or access is severely limited. In fact, Poblenou was the first superblock, created in 2017 by the city government as an attempt to take back the city from cars. It was enormously controversial at the time, as businesses feared the loss of customers and residents worried that they would lose access to cars, transportation, and curbside parking.[20] The neighborhood divided, with factions emerging and residents hanging pro- and anti-superblock banners from their balconies. With local groups gridlocked, the city government decided to sneak the changes in when most residents were away on August holiday, presenting residents with a fait accompli when they returned tanner and a bit calmer. The vacation glow may not have survived the new bollards that blocked traffic, but seven years on, it's hard to see what people were so worked up about. A few cars make it through designated cross streets, but the nine blocks of Poblenou are owned now by pedestrians. In Poblenou and the other superblocks of Barcelona, the streets are alive with foot traffic, shouts of the playground, and the casual mingling of the generations that has made Barcelona such a cultural magnet in the first place.

Design plays an important, but largely overlooked, role in social connection and intergenerational relationships. In Singapore, the design of Kampung Admiralty has put seniors in the middle of the community. In Barcelona, the creation of superblocks, though far more limited than originally envisioned, has taken people out of their cars and put them on street level. It is difficult, virtually impossible, to build relationships with people who whiz by in cars. The idea of the superblock is to coax people out of their homes into an environment that is conducive to conversation, chance encounters, and social connections. It is an idea that has been increasingly lost in modern, urban society—the loneliness of the big city—and it's particularly worrisome in Spain, where family and neighborhood have been the source of emotional and physical sustenance for generations. In Bilbao, just two days before, I was struck by how everyone was living outdoors and communally: Cafés were filled from morning to night, and the sounds of the city were not cars but the clink of cutlery, laughter, and shouts of anguish as Athletic

Bilbao went down once again to Atlético Madrid. Even the region's famous snacks, the pintxos, named after the toothpicks that hold them together, are bar foods designed to be eaten with one hand so that you can drink, gesture, or hug with the other. I'm not going to say that bars are the key to healthy longevity—jamón serrano, blood sausage, gelato, and lots of day drinking and smoking are enough to make a cardiologist curl into a ball—but the communal nature of life in Bilbao, the social connections that are being forged, the fact that you can't enjoy it without getting out of the house, is certainly a piece of the puzzle.

Barcelona, a much bigger, more sprawling city, has long been at risk of losing these social connections so critical to health, belonging, and culture in Spain. Depending on who you ask, it's the fault of cars, or rising housing prices, or the hordes of tourists who unload at the port, or more likely some combination of them all, but it is widely perceived that the soul of the city is gradually disappearing, and with it the health of the community and its residents. Superblocks allow people of all generations to meet in the streets once again, hang out at the cafés, or simply sit side by side on a bench in companionable silence. They may be friendships of a lifetime, or casual acquaintances renewed fitfully, but they are the stuff of villages, not cities, and they can be a critical part of the infrastructure of social connection and healthy aging.

———

Using housing and design to bring the generations together is a critical part of the Queenstown strategy, but by no means is it the only part. I saw that over a game of mah-jongg at Queenstown Secondary School. Mah-jongg is a fascinating game, not because of the rules, I haven't the faintest idea what any of the players are doing, but because every time I've seen it played—both in real life and in television and movies—it is the exclusive province of old ladies, usually older Chinese women but sometimes older Jewish women who popularized the game in the US in the middle of the last century. Mah-jongg is a great social game because people talk constantly while playing, and research has even shown that the combination of rapid tile movements and the use of fine motor skills has therapeutic value for older people.[21] If you asked me for an ideal table game for older people, I might say mah-jongg, except that it seems so exclusionary to younger generations less familiar with the game.

Or is it? Because the game I am watching has both demographically typical players (two women in their seventies) and two thirteen-year-olds. The kids are as confused as I am, even as the older players whisper advice to them. I think the older players are taking it easy, but still the tiles move with stunning speed, as if the women had been trained as three-card monte dealers. A round of mah-jongg usually takes about ten minutes and a full game about two to three hours, but this one is over in five minutes. It reflects a huge skill gap between the players, but none of it stops the group from enjoying the experience together.

It's all part of the plan in a trigenerational class at Queenstown Secondary School (roughly equivalent to an American high school) that brings together high school students, college students, and older adults. It's the brainchild of Lynette Tan Yuen Ling, the director of studies at one of the residential colleges at NUS. The program is yet another piece of the Queenstown plan to unite the generations and create mutual support. It is intended to create connective tissue between the generations as part of the overall goal of enhancing health among the district's aging population. "You could be in good health. But if people treat you like you're old and exclude you from everything, your health just goes downhill. . . . One of the critical levers to stop ageism is intergenerational bonding," she says.

It's often expressed to me during my week in Singapore that many feel the loss of generational connections that existed when multigenerational families typically lived together, a system that has gradually declined even as many families continue to live near one another within the tight confines of the country. It hasn't necessarily undermined cultural values of generational respect, but they are more abstract now, and there are fewer opportunities for intergenerational sharing. The trigenerational program, and many others like it, is intended to re-create intergenerational sharing as an everyday activity.

Even though they lose, quite badly as best as I can tell, at mahjongg, it's the youngest students who are the drivers of the trigenerational project. On the day that I attend the class, small teams from the secondary school are presenting their plans to foster intergenerational cohesion. The first group proposes a "Jenerational Jam," suggesting the team's fascination with alliteration if not spelling. The team leads us through a series of shared activities, including mah-jongg, chair Zumba (less of a hit since the younger participants seem to be rather confused by the macarena . . . I dig it, though) and scrapbooking. Food is a great uniter of generations: One team demonstrates intergenerational cooking while another pushes a dessert taste test between traditional foods and more modern confections. I worm my way into being appointed a judge and pronounce the strawberry cheesecake superior to the tutu cake. Chalk one up for modernity.

There is an emphasis on alternating activities that are familiar to the elders with those that are comfortable for the students. After mah-jongg, two groups square off over a game of virtual bowling, much to the delight of the kids. It's pretty forgiving, more strikes than anything else, but enough gutter balls and balls lifted straight into the air to remind us that not everyone is fluent with digital games. But it's all good-natured as the class applauds the strikes and merrily jeers the gutter balls. I'm not sure how many of the students are going to master the recipe for Aunty Poh Lin's egg fried rice or understand the subtleties of mah-jongg, and it seems unlikely that the elders are going to become foosball masters anytime soon, but that's not the point really. It's to spend time together, gain familiarity, and build relationships, and especially for the elders, have some productive fun—something astonishingly valuable to our health and well-being.

Intergenerational activities are everywhere in Queenstown. Even the senior centers are being infused with intergenerational principles. And it's not just the existing active aging centers but also new organizations, like Ibasho, that are reinventing the field. Ibasho was created by Emi Kiyota, now a professor at NUS but somewhat of a pied piper for intergenerational cohesion who has bounced from Japan to the United States and now to Singapore, where Wong has recruited her to help spread the good word. Ibasho defies easy categorization: It's a senior center, but one that embraces participation by younger people. Ultimately, the goal of Ibasho is to create a place where the "young learn from the richly lived lives of older people and the elderly learn from the young's ability to pick up new things quickly."

By happy coincidence, the first Singaporean Ibasho center was opening that very morning in Queenstown. Despite the lack of any real advertising or concerted effort to promote the first exercise class, more than two hundred people showed up for the first session, though most had to be turned away as the room could only accommodate seventy. I miss the opening ceremonies, but I return later that day to meet with the new Ibasho steering committee. Like the place itself, the committee is age-diverse. Jason, age thirty-four, rocks his infant son in his arms as he tells me about his attention to connecting the generations. He dates his interest in intergenerational activities back to his own close relationship with his grandfather, first as a care recipient from him and later as a caregiver for him. But Jason is not even close to being the youngest member of the steering committee. The youngest is age nineteen, just out of polytechnic high school, and not at the meeting today as he is on a job hunt, but his very place in the organization reflects the central conceit of uniting generations for everyone's benefit.

———

I suspect that some readers may be thinking, "Well, that's Singapore," with the implications that the lessons from there may not be transferable to larger, more diverse, and less managed societies like the US, the UK, or pretty much anywhere else. There is some truth to that; all countries are different, and Singapore is more different than most. Singapore's global image is shaped to a certain extent by its unusual preoccupation with cleanliness (the sale of chewing gum is forbidden and littering is severely punished), its stunning architectural assemblies such as the Marina Bay Sands Hotel and the Interlace, and its continued use of severe physical punishments such as caning, leaving for some the impression that the country is some type of authoritarian wonderland. William Gibson's acid description of Singapore as "Disneyland with the Death Penalty" is amusing in a condescending kind of way, but it does vividly capture Singapore's unique mix of economic exuberance and political and cultural conservatism. And Singapore is tiny, wealthy, and centrally controlled in ways few countries are.

That all may be true, but it fails to recognize, as most critiques of Singapore do, the underlying source of the country's success. Singapore since its inception has been a welter of contradictions— Chinese, Malay, Indian, and English; businesses and unions; native-born and foreigners—and a form of paternalistic single-party rule has survived, and remained popular, because the government has proven adept at forging consensus among these competing and sometimes hostile groups. Progress in Singapore is not simply the result of government fiat and wealth, but of all of society having committed to long-term planning, consensus building, and certain cultural values such as the importance of educational attainment and familial support. It may be that those values are difficult to import in an age of cultural dissonance, but it is certainly worth trying if the payoff is better health and better social outcomes.

In fact, while the focus on intergenerational relationships may have reached its full flower in Singapore, it is by no means unique to it. Of all the issues I researched, the focus on intergenerational relationships and their centrality to social connection, purpose, and health was the most universal one across all five countries that I visited for this book. Ibasho itself started in Japan, and there are other Ibashos, whether they know it or not, in cities around the world.

Bergamo in Northern Italy is one such place. By all rights, the town should be known for its wonderfully preserved Città (High Town), cobblestoned streets, lovely cathedral, and the endless set of stairs leading up from the lower town that left me terribly sweaty and unpresentable for my meeting with the mayor, Giorgio Gori. But in this decade, Bergamo is best known as one of the epicenters of the COVID-19 pandemic, the first city outside of China to feel the full brunt of the disease. For weeks, Bergamo was the virus's playground as it romped through homes, schools, and hospitals, with deaths so frequent that the city's overworked priests had to quiet the tolling of the bells for the dead.[22] Tourists and residents deserted the town square, only to be replaced by the klieg lights of CNN and other broadcasters seeking to tell the story of this horrifying and deeply mysterious plague.

The majority of the early victims in Bergamo, as in most places worldwide, were older, and you might think that the resulting strategy after the COVID-19 pandemic would be to keep older people farther apart, bubble-wrapped from the potential infections of daily life. But Bergamo has gone in exactly the opposite direction, believing that social isolation was a cause of fragility and that greater integration and cohesion will lead to a healthier, more resilient population. As a first major step, the city is transforming its entire network of senior centers into "Centers for All Ages," part of a strategy to reintegrate the generations and build social capital for older adults. Senior centers are a well-developed system in Bergamo, operating in each of its twenty-two neighborhoods. Out have gone the cards and Bingo (I'm sad, I love Bingo), and in have come dancing and music, cultural excursions, theater, classes developed by the University of the Third Age, after-school activities, tutoring of the young by the old, and tutoring of the old in digital literacy by the young. It's a vision of an integrated community center and a transformation of Bergamo from an age-segregated city into an intergenerational village.

———

Singapore may be the model for intergenerational integration, but Italy is not that far behind. The fact that the Italian effort is more local, less organized, and less uniform says more about the character of civic efforts in Italy than the nature of the commitment. Italians will tell you that this less centralized approach will allow for more innovation and experimentation, and whether you want to credit that as a general concept or not, it certainly is the case in Udine.

Like Bergamo, Udine is a postcard-perfect town that Northern Italy seems to stamp out with appealing regularity. I'm not there to sample the charms of a city known for its gracious plazas and inviting cafés, but instead to understand the Playful Paradigm, the city's unique approach to social and intergenerational connection. Beginning in 2010, the city, wrestling with the increased social isolation of its rapidly aging population, developed the project on the theory that games and play—and fun in general—would bring elders out of their homes and knit the generations together. The locus for this effort is the Toy Library. It is an evocative name, and there are certainly toys there, especially on the first floor where the small children have dominion. But as you ascend to the second and third floors, the toys turn into games, mostly board games, designed to bring intergenerational groups and families together around a table. I visit at midday, a time when the library is typically closed, but in a few hours, the rooms will brim with young and old, families and singles, because the Toy Library has become a convening point in the city.

The games don't stop at the edge of the library. We walk outside to the attached pocket park, where teenagers are playing on the giant chessboard and the black queen is threatening the white king, much to the dismay of the team that even at a quick glance seems certain to lose. Every park in the city has games like the giant chessboard that are intended to turn solitary activities into collective ones. And if you are not near the library or a park, or if you want something else, the city provides the Ludobus, literally "the toy bus," which travels around the city bringing games and toys to children of all ages, sort of like Santa in a minivan.

Over the years, the Playful Paradigm has become the organizing principle for numerous city services and city festivals in Udine.[23] The biggest events of the Udine social calendar are Pi Day (March 14), the annual Energy in Play fair, and World Games Day. On Pi Day, the city closes its streets at 4:00 p.m. so that people can enjoy the math games and pi-related challenges, but also eat, dance, and sing— perhaps what you might expect from a program that emphasizes fun, play, and social connection as a core strategy for public health.

The Playful Paradigm has spawned imitations in cities ranging from Dublin, Ireland, to Klaipeda, Lithuania. Play is a delightful organizing principle, and there is, in fact, well-regarded research demonstrating that games are among the most effective leisure activities, better than even reading or playing a musical instrument, for staving off cognitive decline, likely thanks to the combination of mental challenges and the social opportunities created.[24] But research aside, let's just say that building an entire social health platform around play is unusual, even idiosyncratic, and I press Stefania Pascut, who runs social services for the city, to tell me how Udine got into the games business in the first place.

Stefania demurs to what I think of as a rather straightforward question. Instead, she offers to call Furio Honsell, pulling out her mobile to see if the former mayor can make an impromptu appearance at the Toy Library. I can't say that I was terribly keen for the extra interview. I knew Honsell had been mayor of Udine when the city launched the Playful Paradigm program, but elected officials often make for lousy interviews either because they are conditioned to talk at length without saying much, or they don't have enough programmatic knowledge to be terribly useful. But I took solace in the belief that it was unlikely Honsell, now a member of the provincial council, would drop everything to talk with an obscure foreign writer.

Twenty minutes later, I hear him clomping up the steps of the Toy Library. In his mid-sixties, Honsell is short and bespectacled with a tidy graying beard and mustache. If anything, Honsell looks like a college professor, which is understandable because he previously taught computer science at the University of Udine before becoming its rector in 2001. Pascut introduces us, and mere seconds later Honsell has reached into the sack he is carrying to show me his favorite games. The bag is full of them: modern games, games from the Renaissance, puzzle games, board games, sleight-of-hand games, and mathematical tile games that I can't quite follow. I may not have understood all of Honsell's games, but it's easy to see that the man just loves them. Forty-five minutes on, Honsell has worked his way through the entire sack of games (except one that apparently requires me to wear a suit jacket, which I have eschewed on an unseasonably warm spring day), shown me the games column that he writes for a national economic publication, and offered me the secret of his success at Wordle, which he plays in four languages every day. It may not sound that great to you, but his genuine enthusiasm for the topic makes for a charming and revealing conversation. And it answers my question: Because of his own passion for games, Honsell immediately saw the link between gaming and social connection, so when he became mayor, it was not a large leap to think of games as a tool for bringing people together to promote and foster healthy aging.

The case for intergenerational connection is built on a very solid foundation of research, but one of the things that I learned during my travels is not to discount the importance of personal passion in creating effective intergenerational programming. It's one of the reasons that music is such an effective and meaningful mechanism to bring the generations together. If you want to feel that lump in your throat, show up for a performance of the intergenerational drum corps at St. John's-St. Margaret's Church in Singapore, and see the seniors from the nursing home, all in wheelchairs, and the tiny students of the adjacent preschool pound away with great enthusiasm, if not great skill, on overturned plastic buckets. Or go to the annual "Threads" concert at the Kursall Congress Centre in San Sebastián, Spain, where intergenerational choir groups from all over the province come together to share the stage, sing songs, play instruments, and to culminate the show, offer a heartfelt rendition of the Threads Anthem.

Or if you happen to find yourself in Salamanca, Spain, home to the second-oldest university in Europe, tune in to "Tuna," the name used universally (for reasons I have not been able to track down) by college singing groups throughout Spain. I'm listening to this Tuna at the opening dinner for the Spain-Japan Summit on Longevity (yes, that's a thing). Its twenty singers and guitar players are all men and all wearing Renaissance-era robes festooned with patches commemorating their past singing events and competitions. The Salamanca Tuna dates back to medieval times when poorer students had to sing for their supper—and tuition. But more importantly for my purposes, the Tunas are what I would call a naturally occurring intergenerational activity. Once a Tuna, always a Tuna. Unlike the other college groups that I am familiar with—though my knowledge is hardly encyclopedic on that topic—the group includes current students, recent graduates, and much, much less recent graduates, as the age of the group members ranges from roughly twenty to approaching seventy, with numbers evenly distributed across the generations. It's a seemingly ageless environment with roles and responsibilities divided without reference to hierarchy, seniority, or any rule of incumbency. The fact that the Tuna group flourishes as an intergenerational activity without ever thinking of itself as one makes it all the more meaningful and effective.

———

I feel the same specialness the moment I leave the streets of Kanazawa in western Japan and walk into the spacious, welcoming halls of Bussi-En. For some, that specialness might be the working Buddhist temple that abuts the front door, or it might be the stream that runs through the main building. But for me, it is one of the first conversations in the building, as Hiro and I are getting a tour of the facility before our interview with Bussi-En's founder, Ryosei

Ohya. As we pause near the café, our guide briefs us on how it is run exclusively by older adults and young people with Down syndrome. One of the servers, a young boy with Down syndrome, walks into our conversation. He doesn't join, at least in the ordinary sense, but rather walks into our tight circle, peering up at each of us as if we are a piece of art to be examined and discerned. In other settings it might have been discomforting, mostly because it is hard to know how to react outside the rules of conventional conversation, but no one here bats an eye. It is clear immediately that this is a natural, common, and accepted occurrence, a reflection of the social ethos of Bussi-En—the Gochamaze, or "mixing together," philosophy of the place.

Bussi-En is hard to categorize. Formed around a six-hundred-year-old Shinto temple—Ohya is also the temple priest—the organization encompasses a kindergarten, a spa, a restaurant, a gym, yoga classes, a community medical clinic, a therapy center for Alzheimer's patients, a bar, and the working temple, not least of all. It's a jumble for sure, and it irritates my innate need for orderliness, but Hayami Kenji, who has the opaque title of corporate director and has taken on additional duties as our tour guide, tells us that "society was originally all mixed up. Then we started separating children, the elderly, the disabled. We're just trying to bring people back together."

And that they do. Over a thousand people come to Bussi-En every day, more than half a million a year. They are the young and the old, the disabled, and just neighbors in the community. Roughly a third of the center's visitors come for particular services like visiting the clinic or taking a class, but the majority are drop-ins, here to attend a celebration, to draw on the walls, to hang out at the bar. And it is all mixed up, as Ohya promises. At the café, the workers are old and young, and our waitress has Down syndrome. Upstairs in the lounge, two middle-aged men, wearing the suit and tie of businesspeople everywhere, lean in on their conversation while teenagers cavort on the adjacent sofa, preening when I stop to take pictures of the multigenerational and slightly askew scene.

Ohya tells me that one of the organizing principles of Bussi-En is ikigai—I get my third lecture in two days on the subject—and he is particularly attentive to helping older people find purpose and meaning in their aging years. Older people are the lynchpin of the place—not being taken care of but taking care of others. They support disabled colleagues at the restaurant, the gym, and the bar; they help with childcare and after-school programs; and they serve as community guides within Bussi-En. Some of the elders are paid, but others are volunteers, working out of a desire to provide social connection, meaning, and ultimately better health for the members of this community. Kanazawa is a community that has been hit hard by earthquakes and floods—it's even snowing the day we show up, which is not a natural disaster even that late in the spring, but perhaps a signal that the gods like to play ecological roulette with this part of Japan—and Bussi-En is a symbol of the community's desire to build anew even in an aging Japan.

I ask Ohya why he is so confident that all the activities taking place at Bussi-En, a wonderful mash-up connected only by their intergenerational contours, are so good for the health of members, especially the elderly. I expect him to reply with an anecdote, a moving story of a community member. Instead, Ohya switches to presentation mode, displaying one chart after another from research projects in Japan and the United States that show the link between social engagement, purpose, and declines in all-cause mortality. It's impressive, but he then leans in conspiratorially and says to me, "All this research came after we started this place. We knew from the beginning that Gochamaze, this mixing together, would help everyone. Research is just catching up with us."

Three Tips for Healthy Aging

And you can catch up too:

Reconsider generational segregation. For a country that prides itself on being a melting pot, we do a pretty good job of dividing ourselves in all sorts of ways: racially, economically, educationally, and politically. But in some ways, age segregation is more pervasive than those other divisions, in part because it is seen as a socially acceptable and appropriate way of living. Table 23 itself was age-segregated, combining people who didn't know one another and perhaps had nothing in common other than their year of birth. It's a testament to the hold that age segregation has on all of us that everyone, including me, accepted this as the natural order of things.

Americans are more likely to have a friend of a different race than one who is ten years older or younger than they are.[25] It's an arrangement at odds with our cultural history, as well into the nineteenth century in the US (and still currently in many places), age was not a defining factor in who people lived with or socialized with. And why should it be? As Ashton Applewhite observed in her anti-ageism manifesto *This Chair Rocks*, "[p]eople who like NASCAR or archaeology, or poker or tango don't age out of those lifetime interests any more than people stop being drawn to working with kids or rescuing whales or playing the piano."[26] I think we can acknowledge that some differences do exist because of your time of life, but that's hardly a reason for age segregation. Differences enhance relationships and friendships and engender curiosity and learning. Table 23 would likely have had better conversations, certainly not one so stuck on the joys of reading during the day, if we had shaken things up and created intergenerational tables. Only convention, and the wrath of the bride's parents, would have prevented us from doing so.

Consider your housing future. Generativity starts at home, by keeping the generations together or at least nearby. For the last century, Americans have, along with people in the UK and many other countries, struggled with this concept. Urbanization, increased mobility, and the cultural favoritism expressed in *Failure to Launch* have pulled families apart, while cultural norms imported by Latino and Asian immigrants have tended to push them back together.

I know where Table 23 stands on the issue. With one exception, everyone at the table was an empty nester. Though they may have expressed mixed emotions, I doubt whether anyone would have it differently if they could. Beth and I were the lone holdouts, but even that will presumably be called into question in two years when Nate heads off to college.

Not everyone has to live in multigenerational households, of course (unless you are in Singapore), but it is time for Table 23 to reconsider whether this is "the way things should be" or not, because if anything, the disassembling of families is a modern attack on our historical and biological imperatives. The good news is that there are increasing options for people who want to think creatively about intergenerational living. Some of those ideas come from the innovation community, from companies like Nesterly and SpacesShared, a Canadian company that similarly matches students with older adults who have extra room in their homes.

Despite the reluctance of Table 23, multigenerational living is on the rise in the US, growing from a historic low of about 7 percent in 2011 to 26 percent in 2021.[27] Part of the increase was surely due to COVID-19, but the dip after the end of the quarantine was shallower than many observers expected. Economics have changed: Housing is increasingly expensive and inaccessible to many younger people. And culture is changing in an increasingly diverse country as the rising numbers of Latinos and Asians in the US suggest that generativity can be a national, not just an immigrant, norm. Public opinion of these arrangements still teeters—over a third of Americans say this trend is "bad for society"[28]—but social acceptance tends to follow economic necessity. Economic reality may lead to more supportive and varied housing options. Lennar Homes has rolled out a "Next Gen" home for multigenerational families. "Granny flats"—secondary housing units often designed to give a relative both proximity and privacy—have also achieved some popularity, particularly in communities dealing with housing shortages. Not every property will support a granny flat, but the idea reflects a compelling combination of closeness and autonomy. Lots of factors are driving multigenerational arrangements—everything from economics to caregiving to mutual support—and when the people of Table 23 consider their next housing arrangement, they should be considering the prospects for multigenerational living well before they think about retirement and other age-restricted communities.

Embrace the intergenerational workplace. Not everyone at Table 23 is working—I've made a pretty big deal of that fact in this book already—but those who still are have the opportunity to embrace the multigenerational workplace. In many ways, the office is still the most accessible source of intergenerational relationships. Young, middle-aged, and late-stage workers mix together, sometimes in work teams, sometimes in mentoring and reverse mentoring opportunities, and sometimes just around the office water coolers, if such things still exist in our post-COVID world.

To be sure, the opportunity for true connectivity is challenged by hierarchy and power imbalances, and by remote work, but given the demographics of the labor force, the future lies in embracing the opportunities for generativity in the workplace. Some places are better for that than others. About three-quarters of job seekers and employees say they value diversity in their job decisions, and age diversity should be part of that matrix. It is not difficult to find companies that care, at least in some measure, about that topic.[29] There are the three thousand companies that have signed the AARP Employer Pledge, and thousands more have signed equivalent commitments in other countries. It is not the case that all three thousand companies are deeply committed to the rights of older workers, but they form a natural starting point for anyone who believes in and wants to be part of the multigenerational workforce.

Chapter 4

The Tomato, the Asparagus, and the Carrot

I'T'S DAMP AND cold outside, but from the table on the second floor of the cozy café we have a pleasingly dry view across the churning waters of Lake Orta. The rain, which had started the night before, is still beating down, forcing almost everyone inside. It's not the weather that tourist towns like Omegna generally favor, but from my snug perch, the rain makes it even lovelier: Mists rise from the waters into the green mountains that ring the town, and the winds add a nice frothy cap to the waves that lap gently up to the lip of the lake.

Not so long ago, Omegna was a factory town, a producer most prominently of homewares from brands like Alessi and Lagostina, but in recent years it has evolved into more of a holiday destination, with tourists trundling up from Milan to enjoy the splendid scenery of Lake Orta and the lush mountain valleys that surround it. It is less famous, though, than the nearby village of Orta San Giulio, known for its intact medieval architecture, or San Giulio Island, which contains a lovely basilica, now home to scores of nuns. Over the years, Orta San Giulio has attracted people ranging from Friedrich Nietzsche to Lord Byron. Omegna, on the other hand, seems to delight in its relative obscurity.

Sitting across from me in the café are the asparagus and the tomato, chatting happily about the volunteer group that they lead called Pro Senectute ("For the Elderly"). To my mild disappointment, Marisa (the asparagus) and Mari (the tomato) are dressed normally for women in their late sixties. But they are enthusiastically telling me about a performance put on by the group for local schoolchildren, teaching them about the value of healthy eating. When I later watch the video of the performance, I can't follow the dialogue, it's all in Italian of course, but the children are happily entertained by Marisa and Mari, Sergio (a cabbage with a German accent), and Claudia (the villain, Candy). The play, I predict, won't make it to Broadway, or whatever the Italian equivalent is, but it will make it across town since it was sufficiently popular to win a promotion from Pro Senectute's hand-hewn outdoor stage to Omegna's main theater.

Omegna is located in the Verbano-Cusio-Ossola province, about 100 kilometers north of Turin. If you take the wrong turn out of town, you'll be in Switzerland faster than it takes the vegetables to vanquish Candy. The area is both healthy and wealthy, with a higher ratio of older people than the rest of Italy, a function of high life expectancy and plunging birth rates. Historically, the provincial government has responded to the rising numbers of older people by trying to increase the supply of nursing homes and bolstering in-home caregiving services. Pro Senectute, an offshoot of a larger national group, was born of a different impulse: the desire to decrease the need for such services by getting elders out of the house and keeping them active, engaged, and healthy, thereby reducing the costs, Marisa tells me with some pride, to the regional government.

They are an energetic bunch. Omegna is small, barely a city, but this chapter of Pro Senectute has carved out a national reputation for the range of activities it has built on a shoestring budget. Among the many programs here in Omegna are regular excursions and hikes, a lovely intergenerational community garden worked by the young and old together, and a new senior clubhouse that holds regular events, including memory games, card games, socializing, and today, interviews with a wandering writer. And it's not just limited to traditional senior activities. If you are looking for music and dancing classes for dementia patients or youth basketball programs, Pro Senectute of Omegna has something for you.

But perhaps the most interesting thing about this group of semi-retired volunteers is their profound appreciation for intergenerational activities. With a modest grant from a local foundation, Pro Senectute has built a playground that mixes children's toys with senior exercise equipment. Activities regularly connect schoolchildren with the elderly, and during the COVID-19 pandemic, the group organized a program for high school students to talk on the phone every week with quarantined elderly residents of Omegna and its surrounding villages.

I'm always game to talk about programs that help older adults stay active, engaged, and healthy, and it's a pure bonus that there are intergenerational elements at work. But here I'm more interested in the volunteers than I am in the program itself, because Pro Senectute is fundamentally a story of older people in service to older people and how that promotes social connection, purpose, and healthy aging for both sides of the equation. Marisa, the asparagus stalk and head organizer of the Omegna chapter, is sixty-eight, and she fits neatly into the demographics of the volunteers. In fact, sitting with a cluster of volunteers, at sixty-one, I'm the youngest one there, and not by a small amount.

It's a pattern that I see throughout my trip in Italy: the elderly in support of the elderly. Mostly it's the "young old" who are the volunteers. Marisa is a pretty good archetype of the group. She's a retired teacher and now virtually a full-time, though unpaid, staffer at the organization. Fundraising, outreach, and programming are all part of her remit. She laughs ruefully as she tells me that when she was a teacher, she kept a diary so that she could account for all her calls and meetings, and today, she has to do exactly the same thing, except now she keeps her records on a phone rather than in a notebook. For Marisa, volunteering has filled the void left by retirement, providing a new passion and purpose and giving her a new circle of friends, colleagues, and confederates to replace the students, parents, and fellow teachers she no longer sees on a regular basis.

But it's not just the "young old" who volunteer in Omegna, a fact that dawns on me when we reach the Pro Senectute clubhouse, a cramped and dingy office suite that nonetheless feels full of life. We have to drive across town to get there, and Mari, a bubbly Italian-English woman in her late sixties, tosses me the keys to her bright yellow Fiat, nicknamed Buttercup, and invites me to drive. It's been twenty years since I've driven a stick, let alone a car so tiny that I think my head might stick out the roof, but it's a joy: quick, agile, and small enough to squeeze through the tiniest of openings, which are the only kind of openings you get in streets that were originally designed for horse and cart, not lorry and car.

The clubhouse is empty when we arrive, but in short order, about twenty-five people cram into the tiny space. Truthfully, it is a little hard to tell who is a member and who is a volunteer. At the extremes, of course, you can at least make an educated guess. There are quite a few people in their eighties and nineties (the oldest person in the organization is ninety-eight), and I assume that they are members, not volunteers. But in the middle you can't tell the difference, and I'm not sure how much it matters. Everyone is having fun and getting something out of it. The participants are getting social connections, exercise, mental engagement, and a sense of belonging—all things that contribute to healthy aging. And so are the volunteers, along with the sense of purpose and meaning that volunteering typically entails. If the goal is to get people out of the home, create meaningful social connections, and add purpose and health to life, it's a little hard to know who is getting the better deal.

If age is the primary demographic sorter in the room, then surely gender is next. It's all women, 100 percent if you don't count me. Sergio, who leads the basketball program and does a little bit of everything else, had been with us at the café but had subsequently abandoned us for other obligations. The lack of men is certainly notable but also not terribly surprising. I'd encountered similarly gendered groups throughout my trip, along with organizers complaining about how hard it is to get men out of the house to join activities. There is an enormous life expectancy gap around the world between men and women of roughly five years, and in every single country it favors women.[1] There are endless theories about why, from the health value of estrogen that favors women to behavioral issues like smoking, eating poorly, and shooting one another that disfavor men. Research backs up some of them, but it overlooks what seems to be an observable cultural disadvantage for men in later life: They are lonelier, more isolated, and less socially connected.

I immediately peg Anita as a participant, not a volunteer, and I'm half right. At Pro Senectute she is a club member, and a regular one at that. I'm not sure how she got to the clubhouse on this particularly inclement Monday, but most days she rides her bike. That alone is an achievement. At age ninety, Anita is proud of her vigor, telling me about skiing on Mont Blanc until she hit eighty and the hiking and climbing that she still does to this day. The outdoor life, and her family, have been the foundation of Anita's life and health ever since she got married at age twenty-one, but she has broadened her interests and activities since her children left the house. She participates regularly in Pro Senectute activities, playing cards, making new friends, and enjoying the group excursions. We thumb through pictures together of a recent trip to local churches, the photos showing both the churches and the visitors wearing their years well. For Anita, the group makes her "feel free." And while she is a member at Pro Senectute, she is also a volunteer in a local nursing home where she goes weekly to "talk with the old folks," a rather daring statement from someone who is likely older than most of the people she helps. But the irony of it all doesn't deter Anita, as the volunteer work gives her a meaning and purpose that was lacking in her now long empty nest.

Volunteering, for Anita, is just one element of a well-rounded, fulfilling life. For her, the family meal, even as her children have moved out of the house, remains a central organizing theme of her week. Once or twice a week, she hosts ten to twelve people—children, grandchildren, great-grandchildren, nieces and nephews—for a family supper, with people arriving in late afternoon and not leaving until eleven or midnight. Anita describes to me with great detail how she makes gnocchi with a Bolognese sauce, which is her treasured recipe. It is a point of pride that her grandchildren and great-nephews have traveled the world and visited the finest restaurants and swear, according to Anita, that her gnocchi is still the best of all.

You don't have to be from a big Italian family to picture the event. Family and food form a cultural core of Italian life—just watch *The Bear* or *The Godfather* if you don't believe me—and the social connection engendered by large, multigenerational, and closely knit families is one of the reasons for Italy's strong health profile. Italians have one of the longest life expectancies and healthy life expectancies in the world despite rather mediocre data on income, smoking rates, and obesity rates—but that is balanced by the high rates of social connection and mutual support. But the centrality of the large family in Italian life is under demographic duress, as birth rates have plunged in Italy to among the lowest in the world, and here in the Piedmont region the rates are even below the Italian average.

But Anita's story shows that the family dinner, especially one built on a firm foundation of gnocchi, has continued to thrive despite the demographic dive and may be buttressed by broader definitions of family to include even more cousins, nieces, nephews, and maybe even those not related to you in the traditional sense. I had seen as much the night before on arrival in Omegna. Hungry from a long drive, fueled only by a few too many Mars bars, I dumped my bags at my hotel and wandered off in search of a nearby restaurant. I quickly found an inviting-looking trattoria, though the owner seemed somewhat puzzled over what to do with a solo diner. Eventually, after some head-scratching and shouting at waiters—and some rather open skepticism about why someone would be eating by himself—he offered me a table tucked into the back corner of the restaurant. I usually don't care if I have a "good" table or not, but this one was so awkwardly placed that it was hard for the waiter to reach me, a defect if you are trying to get something—say, food or drink—from him. But it had an upside: The table afforded me a fine vantage point of the cacophony around me. In front, slightly to my left, was a family of seven: two parents, one grandparent, four children, all carrying on at great volume. I remember with great clarity that when Nate was younger, the goal at any restaurant was to get out without any damage and as quickly as politeness and service times would allow. But this family was here when I arrived and still there when I left, replicating Anita's expansive dinner hour in the restaurant setting.

Opposite them and slightly to my right was a group of eight older friends, all around seventy-five or so. The years had not diminished their enthusiasm for food and camaraderie—or the habit of speaking at rather high volumes. It wasn't a traditional family unit, of course—my guess was that no one was related other than the couples—but you might call it a family of choice. On that Sunday evening, it was filling in for the traditional Sunday dinner that holds such a central role in Italian social iconography.

Culturally, Italians remain far more committed to human connections than Americans. One of the great risks to social connection right now is the internet and social media, and Italians simply spend less time online than others, about three hours per day. The Brits and the Japanese both spend about four and a quarter hours, and Spaniards are online about five hours and forty minutes, but that's nothing compared to Americans, who spend about seven hours a day online, or South Africans, who spend nine and a half hours every day online, or Nate, who would spend twenty-five hours a day online if he could figure out a way to slow the rotation of the earth.[2] Much of the difference in available time is invested in social relationships: with family, friends, and neighbors. Meals play a big role in that time allocation. Italians spend on average ninety minutes at meals every day, compared to just forty-eight minutes for Americans, and they invest some 30 percent more time every day in family, household, and care responsibilities, despite the decline in family size.[3] It suggests to me that Italy will continue to do better than other countries like the US and the UK with social connection even amid demographic change.

———

If I had shown up in Omegna thirty years ago, I would have certainly found evidence of the big family dinner, but I wouldn't have found such a central role for volunteerism and nonprofit organizations in the life of the community. Unlike the United States, which has a long history of volunteerism—Ben Franklin started the first volunteer fire department in Philadelphia in 1736—Italy has virtually no such tradition. For most of the history of Italy and its regional predecessors, the Catholic Church held an essential lock on social services, and it wasn't until the 1890s that reformers seeking to reduce its influence managed to break the monopoly, though even that was in favor of government social programs, not private volunteer organizations.

For the next century, the Catholic Church and the state shared responsibility for virtually all social activities, with the government often outsourcing work to church-related organizations.[4] It was only in the late 1990s, largely in response to government spending cutbacks, that volunteer organizations began to form in significant numbers to plug the emerging gaps in social services.

By 2003, about 826,000 volunteers donated their time to 21,021 voluntary organizations. That may seem impressive, and it certainly is compared to roughly zero just a few years before, but it still represented less than 2 percent of the adult population, a number that paled in comparison to countries such as the United States, Norway, the Netherlands, and Canada. But over the last two decades, the deepening crisis of the Italian welfare state has ignited an entirely new philanthropic third space; there are now an estimated 359,574 charitable organizations in Italy, and by some estimates, over 20 percent of Italian adults volunteer their time.[5] To a certain extent, the rapid growth of the nonprofit sector in Italy is a reaction to austerity within the national government and a deliberate attempt to "marketize" social service functions. To facilitate that transition, the Italian government has enthusiastically supported the expansion of the nonprofit sector, first in 2014 by endowing a five hundred million euro investment fund to spur the creation and expansion of new nonprofits and social enterprises, and then two years later with the formation of a new regulatory scheme by the Italian parliament to encourage the launch and expansion of nonprofits.[6]

More importantly, the change in the regulatory environment has been matched by a change in the cultural context, with more and more Italians associating volunteering with social connection, community belonging, and vitality and health.[7] And that cultural shift has registered most heavily with older Italians. Adults between the ages of sixty and sixty-four now represent the largest percentage of volunteers, a figure that will undoubtedly continue to grow as the number of older adults increases, as the physical capacity of older adults in Italy continues to expand, and as more and more people associate volunteering and a purposeful life with good personal health. In all, it's an extraordinary shift in just a few decades, from a culture that relied almost entirely on government and church largesse to one of the most active and vigorous nonprofit sectors in the world.

"Our goal in Bolzano is to have people dying while they are making love." That comment from Carlo Librera, the head of social services in Bolzano, draws laughter and scorn from his colleagues around the table. I love it, though—it's by far the most Italian thing anyone has ever said to me. But to be fair to Librera, whose towering shock of white hair makes him look more like a German composer than an Italian civil servant, his comment fairly captures social policy here in this midsize city in the South Tyrol, just fifty miles away from Italy's border with Austria.

Most social services agencies focus on the frail elderly: Meals on Wheels, caregiving, medical services, and fall alerts, for instance. It's critical work to be sure, but that's not where Bolzano is focusing its efforts. Rather, Bolzano, like Omegna, has a strategy of helping people age better so that they will never need these services in the first place, so that they can keep doing what they love the most (which can include other things than having sex, as Librera hastily adds) to the end of life. It's not merely rhetoric. It's law in the Autonomous Province of Bolzano-South Tyrol, as the regional assembly has enacted a unique law enshrining active aging as the core strategy of the province.

Active aging has been a fixation for Bolzano, both the city and region, for years. It may be the call of the mountains, we're nestled into the rocky embrace of the Dolomites, and hiking and climbing are a feature of life here. Renzo Caramaschi, the mayor of Bolzano, pops into our meeting to make that point. He's practically a walking commercial for the outdoor life. Even at seventy-eight, he is a picture of vigor, a mountaineer and hiker, the kind of guy who might invite you to punch him in the stomach so that you can test his steely abs. He tells me that he wants to come visit the United States so that he can climb the Rockies. I'm not exactly sure what Rockies he means, they stretch three thousand miles across the US and Canada, but he looks like he could climb them all if he had the time. Caramaschi confidently proclaims that he will summit the Rockies as a ninetieth birthday gift for himself. I don't doubt it.

Volunteerism plays a central role in active aging in Bolzano. Brigitte Waldner, who directs the social and elderly services for the entire province of South Tyrol, tells me that there are 150,000 people who volunteer in the region, out of a total adult population of under 450,000. It's an astonishingly high number, the highest percentage in the nation, but Waldner chalks it up to the German virtues of organization and commitment and the Italian love of community.[8] This mixing up of cultural virtues is an upside, I suppose, of being part of a region that has been traded back and forth between countries and empires for the last seven hundred years.

"Move, move, move" is the core of the active aging strategy in Bolzano, but it's much broader than encouraging everyone to go climb a mountain. The public law starts with the idea that retirement is a career—a remarkably forward-looking way of thinking about it—and needs to be attacked on an individual level with purpose and passion. Part of the role of the government is to fund projects to help retiring people identify that new purpose once work is in the rearview mirror and family has started to spread apart. For years, Bolzano offered a course called "Finally I'm Retired. I'm Rethinking My Life," which captures the notion that retirement is just the beginning of a new and productive stage of life.

Encouraging seniors to attend cultural events is also a piece of the Bolzano strategy. Music, dance, and theater are all underwritten generously by the government, not just in the major cities but in smaller towns that have less regular access to cultural activities. Everyone is encouraged to attend, of course, young and old alike, but there is a focus on getting older people engaged with cultural events—both as volunteers and attendees.[9] Tickets are heavily subsidized, "virtually free" for senior citizens, as is transportation to and from events. And cultural events have been rebranded to get people thinking about the health value of social events. "Culture makes the life longer," a tagline in the city, is presumably a reference to healthy longevity and not the interminable nature of opera.

In the home of Verdi, Puccini, and Rossini, perhaps it's not surprising that the government is so encouraging of opera and other cultural undertakings, but the strategy in Bolzano is actually more Swedish than Italian. Librera tells me that the idea began to coalesce only after a visiting Swedish researcher shared data that showed a connection between attendance at cultural events and declines in all-cause mortality. And it's true: A thirty-six-year study of more than three thousand Swedes, the latest in a long line of research on the subject, found a significant connection between regular attendance at cultural events and life expectancy, even after holding constant for relevant behavioral factors, like smoking, and demographic factors, such as education and wealth.[10] And it's not a small difference: Participants with the lowest level of attending cultural events had a more than threefold higher all-cause mortality rate than those with the highest level of cultural event attendance. It's another example of the epigenetic effects of social engagement: Environmental enrichment such as this can strengthen memory, processing, and overall cognitive health and can lead to reductions in chronic disease.

These are some of the same mechanisms that support the positive health effects of volunteering. There are hundreds, maybe thousands, of nonprofit organizations in the South Tyrol, funded through the regional and municipal governments. Bolzano, I was dutifully informed, is a wealthy community that taxes heavily (that was conveyed with a mix of both pride and regret), permitting robust funding of the social sector, including support for voluntary organizations. All age groups are represented in the large volunteer base, but people near retirement and in retirement are a particularly large source of talent. That explains why so many of the local organizations specifically focus on older volunteers. "Grandpas and Grandmas," for instance, is an organization that sends volunteers to schools to make sure that children entering and leaving school are safe and cared for. There are at least three organizations in Bolzano that focus on older people taking care of other older people. Typically it is the young old, people in the sixty-five to seventy-five age range, taking care of those who are a decade or two older, but like Anita in Omegna, there are some of the oldest helping others as well.

Bolzano, as it turns out, is a great place to challenge some of our assumptions about aging. That's not just because the mayor plans to chew up mountains into his tenth decade, but also because of new thinking about technology and aging.[11] The Bolzano city government has made a priority of helping older residents adopt health technologies—monitoring and reporting technologies that support aging in place—and volunteer organizations play a critical role in training people on how to use new technologies. You might think that would call for a group of young, tech-savvy volunteers to help the old folks learn these newfangled gizmos. There's some of that, to be sure, and far be it for me to question intergenerational activities like that, but Waldner tells me they have learned that older volunteers are more effective in helping their peers with technology adoption. Young people are often not the most patient technology teachers, and in Bolzano they have discovered that older technology teachers are more tolerant, don't cut corners on explanations, and are more likely to be trusted by other elders. It has better outcomes for the students and provides yet another key opportunity in Bolzano for older people to participate as volunteers and help themselves while helping others.

———

But does volunteering really help with healthy aging? Given what we now know about the role of human connection, meaning, and purpose in healthy life expectancy, it is hardly a stretch to imagine the positive role that volunteering can play in healthy aging. Context matters, of course: Going down to the food pantry once a month is good, going three days a week is better; tutoring a child over Zoom is good, meeting with kids face-to-face at their elementary school is that much better. But as a general proposition, it is hard to imagine much that would be better for your health than a set of regular activities that are highly interactive and personally meaningful.

It's a critical proposition for charitable organizations to persuade older people to volunteer. Older adults have always been an important source of volunteers, given available hours and increasing physical capacities, but their importance has grown enormously in recent decades. Even as overall volunteerism has fallen in the US, the number of older volunteers has grown, with the percentage of total volunteer hours from older people growing from 18.5 percent in 2003 to 28.6 percent in 2021.[12] So it's not surprising that nonprofit leaders have long touted the health benefits of volunteering, claiming that such activities confer social and functional benefits for people as they age. But in truth, for many years there was more hope and sketch work than actual science behind these claims.

That began to change in 1999, when a team at Johns Hopkins University set out to test the health benefits of volunteering in a more scientifically rigorous manner. The Hopkins researchers had been approached by a fledgling organization called Experience Corps that hoped to tap the expertise, wisdom, and available time of older Americans to support their communities.[13] Though Experience Corps was still new at the time, it had an impressive lineage. Experience Corps was the brainchild of John Gardner, who had proposed the idea in a concept paper in 1988. Gardner's name has largely been lost to history by now, but he was a formidable figure who had served administrations of both US political parties at a time when such a thing was still possible. His sprawling career encompassed various governmental roles, including a turn as the secretary of health, education, and welfare in the Johnson

Administration, and he later led the creation of the Corporation for Public Broadcasting and Common Cause, among other organizations. The responsibility for developing Experience Corps fell to a young academic named Linda Fried, now the dean of the Mailman School of Public Health at Columbia University, and Marc Freedman, who would later go on to start and lead Encore.org (now CoGenerate), the leading "second act" organization in the country.

Experience Corps launched in 1996 with pilots in five cities ranging from the South Bronx to Port Arthur, Texas, and a cadre of older volunteers working as tutors in underperforming schools. Unlike many other volunteer programs, Experience Corps from the beginning required a very significant commitment from the adult tutors—fifteen hours a week during the school year—and it was hoped that this type of intensive, mostly one-on-one tutelage would have a transformative effect on academic performance. The early years were promising, and in 1998 the Corporation for National and Community Service (now AmeriCorps) provided funding for expansion of the program.

It was all promising stuff but left open several key evidentiary issues. Probably the most important question was whether the intensive tutoring improved long-term educational performance among the kids (it did), but a close second was the question of the impact of volunteering on the volunteers, all of whom were sixty or older. That was the question the Johns Hopkins team was tasked with answering.

To test that question, the Hopkins team designed a randomized control trial. Volunteers were randomly assigned into two groups, a participant group and a control group. At the beginning of the school year, extensive health, behavioral, and well-being measurements were taken of both groups. The participant group was dispatched to spend the school year with Experience Corps. Members of the control group, on the other hand, were sent off to do as little as possible, with the researchers checking in regularly to make sure that they did not undermine the experimental design by volunteering for some other program.

At the end of the school year, both groups were recontacted and retested, with extraordinary results. The participant group exhibited improved health, increased physical activity, stronger social networks, an enhanced emotional profile, and reduced time in isolating activities like watching television. Participants were healthier and more active than they were at the beginning of the year. Conversely, the health of the control group had deteriorated, in some cases significantly: Strength was down, falls were up, and social networks had shrunk. Put bluntly, and you will hopefully forgive me for being a little ageist in this shorthand language, the participant group seemed younger; the control group acted older. It was compelling evidence that active, committed volunteer work could have a huge impact on healthy aging.

The Experience Corps study uncorked an avalanche of similar research projects. Researchers at Carnegie Mellon University found that older adults who volunteer for at least two hundred hours per year decrease their risk of hypertension, or high blood pressure, by 40 percent.[14] Another study looked at participants in the Foster Grandparent Program, finding that 83 percent of volunteers reported excellent or good health compared to a matched population of nonparticipants, of whom only 52 percent reported similar results. Longitudinal studies of Foster Grandparent participants, in which the volunteers were tested at the beginning of the program and then again one year into it, found positive effects on volunteers' self-rated health, loneliness, social connectedness, and symptoms of depression and anxiety. Almost half (46 percent) of new volunteers measured at the baseline reported improvement in health and well-being at the one-year follow-up. Additionally, 63 percent of volunteers who stated that they "often" felt alone reported decreases in feelings of isolation. Over two-thirds (70 percent) of those who reported five or more symptoms of depression at baseline and stayed in the program reported fewer symptoms at follow-up.[15] And, separately, in a study of nearly six thousand people across the US, recently widowed adults felt considerably lonelier than their married counterparts—until they started volunteering for two or more hours per week.[16]

I could go on, but you get the point: There is now overwhelming evidence that volunteering is good for your health at all stages of life, but particularly for older adults.[17] And these improvements in health are not small ones. The advancements in health that the researchers have found—including around hypertension, cardiovascular disease, cognitive decline, and overall all-cause mortality—are equal to or in some cases better than you could expect to find from intensive nutritional or exercise regimens. It's the real doing well by doing good.

———

It turns out that you can do both well and good in lots of different ways. We are conditioned to associate volunteerism with working with established, legally recognized nonprofits such as Experience Corps. The vast majority of studies connecting volunteering and health focus on formal volunteering, perhaps because it is comparatively easy to research. But informal volunteering—defined as volunteer support not coordinated by an organization involving helping someone outside of your personal household—is in many places of equal significance. It's a hugely undervalued resource—in the US alone over half of adults report helping a neighbor, and 10 percent do it on a regular basis—and it is particularly important in isolated, rural, and underserved communities that lack a critical mass of community organizations.[18] Informal volunteering, research has shown, provides health benefits to the volunteers that are equal to or in some cases exceed those of formal volunteering, which makes sense given the combined values of helping others and also strengthening your own social network.[19] More than virtually any other activity, neighbors helping neighbors can turn a town into a community, a home rather than just a house.

I was thinking about the concept of informal volunteering as I began my first morning in Italy. I was heading south from Naples, where I had flown in the night before, to visit Acciaroli, a town famous for its tight-knit social structure and improbable longevity. The thoughts were a welcome distraction from the chaos of the early morning traffic in Naples. Peeking out from my hotel's parking lot, I could see cars pushing into the intersection from all directions: no signals, no yields, and apparently no rules about who goes next. I gently urge my car forward, hoping for the best. Just a few hours in Italy and visions of returning a smashed-up rental car to the Europcar counter are already dancing through my head. My philosophy in situations like this is that acting like you know what you are doing is almost as good as knowing what you are doing, so I stomp on the gas and push my way into the intersection. It works, and I sail through without incident.

If you were to ask people the secret to Italy's remarkable good health, the volunteer economy would doubtlessly not register. Our understanding of health in places like Italy has been shaped by a Blue Zones narrative that has chalked up extended longevity to good diet and low-stress living. It's not that I disagree with the value of having a healthy diet and reducing stress—that's solid advice—but I am suspicious of the methodology of drawing conclusions from small corners of the world where recordkeeping is at best lax or at worst fabricated. Many researchers now dismiss out-of-hand stories of great longevity in these isolated communities. As one leading European expert told me just before I headed to Italy, "Someone will say they are over 100 just because their neighbor did." It's a form of keeping up with the Rossis that undermines the life expectancy narrative. And even if the claim is true, I'm just not that convinced that a statistical oddity from largely remote and insular communities has much relevance to this book. We are not going to all move to a tiny fishing village on the southern coast of Italy or start behaving as if we lived there.

But that doesn't mean that I'm not going to check it out. Call it journalistic inquisitiveness or academic rigor, or better yet, let's label it for what it is: I'm a complete sucker for a good tale about the Fountain of Youth in general and of colonies of centenarians in particular.

Before she died in 1997, Jeanne Louise Calment, a French housewife, lived to the ripe old age of 122. A quarter century on, Calment is still the only person who has been verified to live that long, but the numbers of people who live past 100 are increasing at stunning rates. There is, in fact, nothing all that statistically special about turning 100 compared to, say, ninety-nine, and the impact on global life expectancy of a few hundred thousand people in a world of seven billion is modest at best. But nonetheless, centenarians hold a special place in the public's fascination with aging and longevity. More than once in my travels, communities have touted the rising number of the super-aged to me as evidence of their healthy lifestyle.

Acciaroli is tiny, a mere two thousand inhabitants, but it has achieved some fame as home to an unusually high concentration of centenarians. In 2016, a team of researchers, headed by Alan Maisel, a professor of cardiology at the University of California, San Diego, caused a stir with a report that Acciaroli was home to "more than three hundred" centenarians. Dr. Maisel attributed this astonishing number to a healthy diet, strong social connections, a favorable climate that supports outdoor activities, and, as he told *The Telegraph* newspaper at the time, to the fact that "sexual activity among the elderly appears to be rampant."[20]

The numbers are indeed impressive, but also on their face absurd. Even Japan, the longest-lived society on Earth, only has about one centenarian for every 1,360 persons, not one in seven as claimed for Acciaroli. And if your town has that many people over the age of 100, it also means that you have equal or more numbers of people aged ninety-five, ninety, eighty-five, eighty, and so on. Do the math and you will find that the entire population has to be over seventy-five if the claim is to be even partially believed. In that sense, Acciaroli is similar to other long-lived communities, including the Blue Zones, where researchers have concluded that the claims of hyper-longevity are more likely to be the result of poor recordkeeping and pension fraud than any special insight into healthy living.[21] I don't mean to entirely discredit the notion that people in Acciaroli may live a long time—Italy is one of the longest-lived countries on Earth, and normal statistical distributions mean that some places will stand out—but it is a reminder to take these types of claims with a grain of salt.

The chaotic traffic in Naples foreshadows my entire two-hour drive south to Acciaroli, which is nestled in the administrative region of Campania. Nature has done a pretty bang-up job here in Southern Italy. The drive hugs the sparkling shore of the Tyrrhenian Sea, curving through sharp mountains that serve as picture frames for the waves pounding against the beaches below. The report card on humans is a little more mixed. The Italian government has built a lovely two-lane highway, one that I would ordinarily enjoy driving as it twists and turns through the mountains, each hairpin revealing the next stunning visage of the waters beyond. The Italian people, however, seem intent on turning the road into some type of Mad Max video game, with drivers weaving wildly through traffic without much bother for the conventions of who drives on what side of the road. The video game designers have added the twist that every type of vehicle known to man is allowed to play, so you can't be certain whether the next vehicular face-off will be with a souped-up BMW sedan, a bicycle, an enormous truck, or a tractor rumbling down one side of the road or the other.

Given the vehicular free-for-all, I was a little surprised, though rather pleased, to arrive at my destination in one piece. I was even more surprised to find out that despite the reckless driving and the lowest rate of seatbelt compliance in Europe, driving fatalities in Italy are low by global standards and even moderate by European standards.[22] Perhaps good luck is the best explanation for the astonishingly high life expectancy in Italy, which now tops eighty-four, and the unexpectedly high traffic survival rate. And maybe that good luck has rubbed off on me, because without incident on the long drive, I crest a final hill and drive gently down a twisting street to the center of Acciaroli.

My skepticism aside, whoever planted the first flag here was onto something. Acciaroli sits astride a lovely natural harbor, and the town climbs steeply away from the water toward a ring of stark, brown hills. The hills form a natural protective bowl, giving the town a sense of privacy and me the completely unwarranted feeling that I have discovered some hidden treasure. As I walk along the small working harbor, the sun shines brightly above a clear blue sky, leavened only by enough clouds to give it character. Houses are modest, and many have not been updated with the conveniences of modern life, judging by the clothes drying from many windows. But you might say that they are $100,000 homes with million-dollar views, as even the most modest are terraced in such a way as to have line of sight toward Spain and North Africa.

I'm on the hunt for centenarians. I don't expect that they will be out in large numbers, perhaps they are too busy having sex, but you have got to figure, if it is one in seven, that the odds are on my side. But no such luck. I see families tunneled into the small sandy beach across from the harbor, and as I walk along the upper town, more families—children, parents, grandparents—join me for a stroll along the street. There are older people for sure, though not a particularly notable number, and I spy far more people in the middle-aged and young categories. There is even a large school group of some eighty or so second or third graders and their chaperones, who rather to my annoyance don't seem to have gotten the message that this is a town occupied solely by the very old.

If you had to pick a town with exceptionally long life expectancy, you probably wouldn't start with Acciaroli. It's a poor town in one of the poorest regions of Italy—per capita income in Campania is less than half of the South Tyrol or Lombardy in the north—and there is no obvious health care support to speak of. Smoking is prevalent, and I've already talked about the driving habits: Even if it doesn't kill you, the stress will surely shave years off your life. And you can talk about the healthy Mediterranean diet all you want, but obesity rates in Campania are among the highest in Italy—almost American high at 51 percent for adults.[23]

Apart from the natural beauty, there is an easy neighborliness to the town. I walk down what passes for the main street, trailing behind a middle-aged man. He may not be the mayor, but he might as well be running for office, greeting everyone on the street by name, a quick chat, a hug, perhaps a small joke. It's a scene played out all over town, as this Saturday afternoon becomes an impromptu block party, with people greeting one another enthusiastically. It's not as if people haven't seen one another lately, given the size of the town, and more likely it reflects the Italian concept of "buon vicinato" (good neighbors) and the importance of neighborliness to civic culture. I have always been fond of the expression that "you can live without friends, but you can't live without neighbors," reflecting the importance of mutual aid in sustaining community. I don't know that you have to choose in Acciaroli between neighborliness and friendship, but it is clear to me, watching people on this brilliant Saturday afternoon, that the idea of neighbors helping neighbors is a key part of the way of life here. I've not been to many of the places that are famous, deservedly or not, for their longevity, like Okinawa or Sardinia, but I imagine they are a lot like this—places of community, connection, and social support. I can't say with certainty even after visiting Acciaroli whether it has a large number of centenarians or not, but it does seem like a town where I would want to stay alive to 100 if I lived there.

It is a little disappointing to come to a town famous for its centenarians and not see anyone over seventy-five. It's like going on safari and only seeing a turkey. Nothing against turkeys, mind you; they're a noble bird, no doubt, and they do wonders at Thanksgiving, but that's not what's on the tourist brochures. If there is a lesson here in Acciaroli, it is that our hope for a Fountain of Youth, our desire to find a way to escape or at least postpone the inevitable, has never really gone away, and has simply been recast into legends decorated with science and social science rather than mysticism or faith.

My own quest was unfulfilled, but there is only so much time you can spend wandering the streets of a small town like Acciaroli before you begin to look uncomfortably out of place. I head back to my car, popping in to buy a bottle of water at a little restaurant where I took my lunch a couple hours earlier. And then pay dirt. It's now well past lunchtime, so only one table is occupied, but it is the owner with an impressively old woman, her face creased with age and a singular determination to eat her soup. I didn't get to see her birth certificate, but I would bet you that African turkey that she was over 100. I lean in to see what she is eating, perhaps that is her personal Fountain of Youth, and am a little disappointed to see that it's the same pasta soup I had earlier consumed, so I'm either in for a few bonus years or nutrition is probably not the singular life source that some may claim it to be. But regardless, I have my centenarian sighting to treasure, even if I came up "about three hundred short" on the total list.

———

Kyung Hi Kim, the head of the School of Future Life at Kyungnam University, parks the car. It's no small feat, given that this part of Suncheon is a warren of densely packed stores. It's the Korea I remember from fifty years ago: busy, entrepreneurial, everyone rushing to and fro. If you don't watch out, you'll get run over by someone hurrying to the future. Our little group—we're joined by a delegation from the Lifelong Learning Institute in Suncheon—navigates a series of tightly packed alleyways, shops piled high with goods and helmed by shopkeepers who watch our little procession with curiosity. We finally turn onto the street that is our destination, and the cityscape changes. This street is newly paved, a little broader than the others, and many of the shops are new, or at least newly renovated. We walk past a salon, a tidy electronics store, and several restaurants, including a few with offerings that diverge from traditional Korean fare. That includes Earl Brown, a pleasant-looking café that features a "New Zealand" brunch consisting of eggs Benedict and bagels, neither of which I associate with New Zealand. Judging from the empty row of tables at the front of Earl Brown, New Zealand cuisine may not have caught on in Suncheon, but to be fair, it's not exactly peak restaurant time at eleven in the morning.

We're heading halfway down the block to the "Interesting Shop," which is wedged in next to a new home goods store and across from an older seafood restaurant that has settled comfortably into its remodeled neighborhood. To all appearances, the Interesting Shop is a typical café, albeit a tiny one, serving a modest menu of drinks and bakery items. But that's really a cover for a new intergenerational volunteer effort. The Interesting Shop is modeled on the

Italian "Café Sospeso" (translated roughly as "suspended coffee") movement, a pay-it-forward idea where patrons buy coffees for others as an anonymous act of charity.[24] It's the same here, except patrons leave money and notes for children from the neighborhood schools to have free coffee, tea, and bread after the end of the school day (the bread is sometimes free and sometimes offered at the nominal cost of 100 won, roughly seven cents). The small, bright shop is plastered with upbeat notes of encouragement from adults and 5,000- and 10,000-won notes left behind so that the children can enjoy their after-school refreshments. In return, the children also leave notes, sometimes of thanks but mostly of dreams, of what they hope to achieve with the rest of the day or with the rest of their lives. Every day, scores of children come to the shop to hang out, read, and engage with the elders who are also seeking community in the Interesting Shop. I had puzzled over the name of the "Interesting Shop," and had largely chalked it up to a translation issue, but when I visited, I realized that the name works because the store's fundamental product is not food and drink but conversation, intergenerational communion, community, and social connection.

In truth, I could have stuck this story in the intergenerational or even the work section of this book—the categorization system here is hardly airtight—but the Interesting Shop is part of a larger effort within Suncheon to spur volunteerism and social entrepreneurship, especially among the burgeoning elder population of the city. Suncheon City is one of those many secondary Korean cities that is struggling against the demographic and economic tide. Combine the country's plunging birth rate with the magnetic pull of Seoul on young people, and you end up with lots of Suncheons—midsize cities that are increasingly bare of people under forty. In response, the city has tried to turn its aging population into an asset, funding older people who want to help younger ones and build a new sense of community. The Interesting Shop is one of those efforts, founded by six retirees who are volunteering their time (and perhaps some of their own money) to create this intergenerational haven.

Park Jun Sok leans forward and tells me, "I'd been retired for six months [from my job as an elementary school principal]. I felt a sense of loneliness, of loss. It was the emptiness of retirement. Working here has helped me regain my sense of self and worth and given me purpose again in life." The other five women sitting with us nod solemnly in agreement. It's a moment of reflection in an otherwise infectiously happy interview. Sometimes, I've found, when you conduct a translated interview, it's like watching a game when the sound is badly delayed. You can see the action, but the fun is already over by the time the words arrive. Not so here. I find myself smiling, laughing, even clapping along with my six interviewees even when I don't know what they are saying.

Wei Young Le, a retired city administrator in her sixties, tells me that volunteering at the Interesting Shop has made her "feel more reconnected, worthwhile, more human. I feel like I have gotten younger." The theme of rejuvenation is consistent across all of the women: They report being told that they "look great" or "look happier" with the underlying implication that the idleness of retirement sapped them of their vitality and vigor. The theme of recaptured youth is hard to avoid: The connections with one another and with the children, and the sense of purpose and accomplishment at the Interesting Shop, have reinvigorated the women and at least forestalled the decline of old age. That formulation of feeling young might draw a side-eye look from ageism advocates—why can't you feel good in your sixties?—but let's grant the notion that volunteering here has engendered good health and vitality.

I point to some of the notes that are pinned to the wall and ask for a translation. They are the wishing well of the children: Win the lottery, go to a concert, marry a handsome man. The women laugh at this last one, and then grow serious. Park tells me that the moments that have stood out the most for her are not on any thumb-tacked bucket list, but when the children begin to understand the concept of paying it forward. She tells the story of Cho In Seo, a fourth grader at the adjacent elementary school who was at first puzzled by the idea of free food and drink. But after his free after-school meal, he left behind 100 won so that the next child could enjoy bread too. Later that evening, he returned with his parents and his brother in tow so they could all share in the intergenerational joy of the Interesting Shop and pay it forward, enabling others to feel that as well.

Formal volunteering is a relatively new, and still undervalued, concept in Korea, a society built around familial self-sufficiency. Even with the push from local governments as in Suncheon City, volunteer rates in Korea remain low compared to the United States and other countries. A 2019 Time Use Survey put volunteer rates among older Koreans at just 6.5 percent, a number that is dwarfed by the US and Italy, for instance.[25] But the numbers are increasing as older Koreans begin to see volunteerism as a route to more personal fulfillment and better personal health.

———

The arrows have generally pointed in the opposite direction in much of the West. Formal and informal volunteer rates in the US have long been among the highest in the world and remain so to this day. It reflects in part different political and social philosophies surrounding the division of responsibility between government and the private sector, with the US counting on the philanthropic and voluntary communities to shoulder a greater portion of civic virtue. And older adults play a significant role in giving both money and time. Controlling for demographic factors, volunteer rates in the US typically fall during early adulthood, then start rising during midlife, increasing until roughly age seventy-five before starting to decline again.[26]

In some ways, the picture of volunteerism in the US remains robust compared to other countries, but starting around 2005, the volunteer rates for Americans in general began a slide that continues to this day. Formal volunteer rates have been tracked closely since at least the beginning of this century, with participation rates peaking among adults in the three years from 2003–2005, and they have steadily fallen since, down about 21 percent over that time. The numbers would be far worse but for older adults, who have bucked the overall trends and continued to volunteer at near-historic rates.

There are many reasons for what has been a significant and long-lasting decline in social participation. COVID-19 certainly played a depressive role, but the decline both predates and post-dates the COVID-19 pandemic. Experts have attributed some of the decline to larger demographic forces. Volunteer participation tends to ramp up when people have children, perhaps because parents feel they have a greater stake in the community, so the fact that more women are delaying childbearing has a dampening effect on overall volunteer rates. And volunteer rates in rural areas tend to be higher than in urban settings, so the depopulation of rural areas has had the dual impact of increasing need for those left behind and driving down total volunteer rates. But underlying the decline is the overall loss of social connection and social capital in the United States. Nathan Dietz, a professor at the University of Maryland and the head of its wonderfully named Do Good Institute, told *The Washington Post* that "[t]he most commonly cited reason why people volunteer, period, is because people ask them to volunteer."[27] As our social relationships have become more distant and attenuated, the interpersonal relationships that drive volunteering in the US have themselves declined and become less effective.

It's similar, even a bit worse, in the UK. Regular volunteering (defined as at least once a month) has declined precipitously from a high of 27 percent in 2013 to only about 16 percent today.[28] The volunteer shortage has crippled any number of charitable organizations, including perhaps most embarrassingly the Big Help Out, a campaign to highlight the value of volunteering that has struggled to stay together because of the lack of volunteers. Even more so than in the US, older people have been the most reliable source of volunteers in the UK, but participation rates among older adults peaked around 2010 and started a slow ebb that turned into a free fall during COVID-19. And recent surveys have suggested that older Brits aren't going back anytime soon—a post-pandemic hangover that will likely have the snowball effect of reinforcing isolation and the loss of social capital among seniors.[29]

It's difficult to make generalizations on a global basis—reporting is episodic at best, and definitions of formal and informal volunteering are inconsistent—but the trends generally are not favorable. They are also not uniformly negative, as the case of Italy proves. In Germany, for instance, to combat the widespread perception that an aging population was a burden on society, the government in the

1990s began to create a national network of Senior Citizens' Offices with the responsibility of supporting volunteer activities by older Germans—and rebranding older people as contributors to society. The federal authorities also reframed volunteering as being healthy for older volunteers, with dramatic results.[30] The project was started with forty-four offices and has now grown to more than five hundred, and volunteer rates among older Germans have almost doubled over the last quarter century.[31]

The experience of Germany highlights the fact that volunteer rates of older people need not rely simply on the promotional efforts of charitable organizations or peer-to-peer networks. More strategic efforts to make volunteering opportunities prominent and easy to access can have a significant impact on volunteer rates. There is irony here. In many places, including the United States, the social sector is seen as an alternative to governmental programming, "a thousand points of light" in the terminology of the White House of George H. W. Bush. But that's not the whole story. Government is by far the largest single source of funding for charitable organizations, and the volunteer sector has in recent decades tended to flourish when government acts as an affirmative partner, providing not only funding but also support infrastructure and public awareness.

You can see that in Singapore. It's not always been easy to imagine a strong charitable impulse in a nation that has cherished what is sometimes locally referred to as the "five Cs": cash, cars, credit cards, condos, and country club membership. But the less-than-fertile environment has not dissuaded Singapore. After the Experience Corps research was released, the government swiftly latched onto volunteerism as an avenue to promote healthy aging, and it launched the National Senior Volunteerism Movement, which includes interlocking programs such as the Community Befriending Program, the Silver Volunteer Fund, and the President's Challenge, all with the aim of increasing volunteer participation by seniors. All of this has resulted in more than a doubling of the volunteer rate among seniors from 13 percent in 2008 to 29 percent in 2016, a figure that now exceeds even that of the United States.

It's hard to miss the connection between volunteering and better health in Singapore. Volunteer efforts are spread across a number of different organizations, but all under the banner of "I Feel Young SG," as if to hammer home the point that volunteering helps older Singaporeans stay vibrant and healthy. Subtlety is not the strong point for healthy aging efforts in Singapore. But accessibility is. At least three government-supported websites—SG Cares, giving.sg, and volunteer.sg—provide easy access to thousands of volunteer opportunities across dozens of different causes. If you want to put your counseling or reading skills to work—or your photography, emceeing, software development, or even "befriending" skills, for that matter—Singapore has a place for you. And if you prefer a less digital experience in signing up, Singapore runs twenty-four volunteer centers around the city to match volunteers with volunteer opportunities.

Singapore (and Germany) have succeeded by making volunteer activities easy to access. The United States is in some ways the opposite situation. There are 1.5 million charities in the US alone, meaning that there is a charity in every community and for every interest. But it also means that the charitable sector is dense, difficult to navigate, and often frustrating to would-be volunteers unfamiliar with the sector. As Germany, Italy, and Singapore suggest, it doesn't have to be that way.

—

Good health habits should start when you're young. That's true for nutrition and exercise, and for volunteering as well: Volunteer rates among older adults are much higher for those who started volunteering during midlife or earlier.[32] Social connection is a little like that as well. It's not that you can't develop important social connections later in life, and much of this book has focused on how to do that, but it's easier if you have built good habits and laid a foundation of relationships earlier in life.

I am reflecting on that fact as I wait for Maria Elisa Ojeda to meet me at a small vegetarian café in center-city Barcelona. She arrives late, out of breath from her ride over on her bright purple bike, which she folds up as we make introductions. It's one of those challenging days for Elisa as she tries to juggle parenting duties with her plan to rent a van and drive to Valencia, some four hours away, to pick up a rickshaw specially adapted to help transport the elderly and disabled by bicycle.

Elisa is the local founder and manager of a nonprofit called, in Catalan, En Bici Sense Edat, which translates roughly to "Cycling Without Age." Originally launched in Denmark, the organization first found a foothold in Spain in Barcelona, and it now operates relatively autonomously in thirty-some cities across the country. Cycling Without Age (I'll default to the English translation) offers bike rides to people with disabilities and the elderly so that they may enjoy the freedom and grace of bicycle outings. If you want to picture it, think of a reverse rickshaw with a bicyclist in back and a two-person carriage in front.

Cycling Without Age is not a transportation project—its primary purpose is not to get people from place to place—but a social connection effort, as Elisa explains it, to enable those with less mobility, particularly the elderly, to get out of the house and talk with the volunteers as they move around the city. When I ask Elisa to tell me what the project provides for its participants, she tellingly starts with the pedalers—not the passengers—and what they learn from the project. She describes what many volunteers, and there are hundreds spread across Barcelona and Spain and tens of thousands across the world, get from the elderly: their ideas, their stories, and new friendships that arise from these excursions. Elisa lights up with laughter as she tells me about one elderly regular who just wants to talk with someone about the Rolling Stones because no one at her senior center is interested, and the volunteers who vie for the opportunity. The organization celebrates the idea of wind in your face, a lovely thought for anyone who has to spend much of their time indoors, but it is less the physical aspects and more the opportunity to forge intergenerational friendships that makes these trips special and coveted. Most people would look at Cycling Without Age and think, "Isn't it great that those nice young people are helping all those old folks." I look at it and think, "Isn't it great that those cyclists, young or old (the oldest volunteer cyclist is ninety), can get the benefit of new social connections, of a greater sense of purpose in their lives, and insights from other generations."

———

Most of the research around volunteerism and health focuses, reasonably enough, on the impact on the individual, but you can also think about it in a broader sense, in terms of what high rates of volunteerism can do for the health of an entire community. One of the most interesting places to see that is in Appalachia, perhaps the unhealthiest region in America. The singer John Denver described Appalachia as "almost heaven," and while that may be a tad exaggerated, it is home to more than its share of America's natural beauty. The Appalachian Mountains form the eastern spine of the US, running 1,500 miles all the way to the Alabama border, and the region is pocketed with craggy mountains, deep valleys, and old-growth forests. The natural beauty is marred, though, by human ugliness—grinding poverty, high rates of drug addiction, and an epidemic of despair—all of which have contributed to a life expectancy that is only 76.9, almost two and a half years lower than the national average.[33]

Virtually every community in Appalachia bears the scars of poor health—most of the shortest-lived counties in the country are concentrated in Appalachia—but there are a few places that defy the gravitational pull of obesity, drug abuse, and suicide. These places are labeled as "bright spots" by the Appalachian Regional Commission, and they overperform in terms of lower rates of chronic diseases, better mental health, and lower all-cause mortality rates. The thing that distinguishes these ten counties (out of 423 in the region) from their neighbors, the commission found, was not income, or access to health care, or diet or exercise, but a culture that supports health and social connection—high rates of volunteerism and a strong social fabric.[34]

I ponder that idea as I look out over the Palazzo Frizzoni from the windows of Bergamo's city hall. Minutes earlier, I'd been ushered up to the reception hall outside the mayor's office. The reception area is large enough, at least tall enough, to hold a basketball court,

with richly tiled floors, ornate mirrors on the walls, and frescoes on
the ceiling. I'm greeted by the mayor's affable spokesperson, Fran-
cesco Alleva, who is wearing an Abercrombie & Fitch sweatshirt
and jokes with me that I have wandered in on casual Tuesday. He's
the only thing casual in the building, as near as I can tell. Everyone
else is in suits and ties, and the artwork ranges from triumphal—an
epic depiction of the Battle of Legnano, the twelfth-century victory
of the municipalities of Northern Italy over the armies of the Holy
Roman Empire—to censorious—an entire portrait gallery filled
with the unsmiling and I can only imagine disapproving visages of
about thirty popes or so.

But I'm not in Bergamo to critique public art (or the fashion
choices of city officials) but to understand how the city became the
national City of Volunteers and a symbol of the changing participatory culture in Italy. It's a surprising designation since until just a
few years ago the voluntary sector in Bergamo was relatively small
and nascent. COVID-19 changed that.

Alleva stares out at the Palazzo Frizzoni with me. I see an
immaculately preserved twelfth-century royal enclave, but Alleva is
reliving the horrors of COVID-19. It's hard to find a silver lining in
the storm of the pandemic, but for Bergamo, Alleva tells me, it was
the emergence of a new civic spirit and a rising tide of volunteerism. Quickly organized as "Bergamo for Bergamo," it began as an
effort to deliver meals, medicines, and other supplies to the many
quarantined, mostly older, residents. As the COVID-19 pandemic
spread and the quarantine deepened, volunteers rushed to make
hundreds of thousands of deliveries of food and medicine across
the town. Many of the volunteers were young, of course, but as the
first days passed, more and more of the healthy old—those with

fewer comorbidities and COVID-19 risks—joined the volunteer ranks. As Alleva described it to me, Bergamo for Bergamo became the centerpiece of the town's recovery effort and a statement that the town would fight and survive the pandemic—and it afforded the volunteers a sense of purpose in a time of despair. The pandemic passed, but the idea of Bergamo for Bergamo did not. Even today, volunteer rates in Bergamo remain unusually high for Italy, especially among the young and among healthy, recently retired people in their fifties, sixties, and seventies. And if Bergamo has its way, they will stay healthy and keep the city vigorous as well.

Three Tips for Healthy Aging

If you want to start volunteering, the good news (and to a certain extent the bad news) is that you will have lots of choices, wherever you are. In addition to the estimated 1.5 million charities in the US, there are four hundred thousand more in the UK, 170,000 in Canada, five hundred thousand in China, and two million in India.[35] These numbers may well include a slice of barely active organizations, but the point is still unmistakable: Wherever you are, there will be options to choose from.

For my friends at Table 23, some of whom have already dipped their toes into the waters of volunteerism, here are some things to consider:

Invest time. Research suggests that the health benefits of volunteering are proportional to the time invested: The more that you put in, the larger the health returns. Experience Corps, at the time of the Johns Hopkins research project, required a time commitment of fifteen hours per week, and the organization, now run by the AARP Foundation, still asks for four to six hours per week as a minimum commitment. You can go still lower: Researchers have tested volunteering at around 100 hours per year and still found significant health benefits in terms of better physical functioning and higher physical activity, beneficial psychosocial outcomes, and lowered mortality rate.[36]

The average American spends about fifty hours a year volunteering, though that number is depressed by the fact that it includes people who work a significant number of hours per week and volunteer on the side.[37] For older people, aged sixty-five and up, who have fewer work commitments as a group, the average time is higher at about 120 hours per year, or roughly two hours per week. By comparison, the average American invests almost six times that on their health and fitness regime every week.[38] If you had to assess the health value of your time, it turns out that volunteering is a much better investment in your own health and that of your community.

Find the right organization. The right organization is the one that you are most passionate about and where you will want to contribute the most time. But not everyone has that passion, at least at the beginning. So where to start when the choices seem endless? Look for places that have established and well-managed volunteer programs, or that allow you to interview first to see if it is a good cultural fit. Check out websites like volunteermatch.com or cogenerate.org to get ideas about volunteer opportunities. And recognize that the first place is not always the right place. Ninety percent of Americans say they want to volunteer, but only 25 percent do, in part because it is often difficult to find an organization that matches

up with schedules and passions or has volunteer roles that are perceived as sufficiently interesting. But with well more than a million
charities in the US, the right match is out there.[39] If you are older,
consider organizations that are specifically designed to leverage the
experience, knowledge, and wisdom of older people: Experience
Corps, Foster Grandparents, and Big & Mini are just a few examples. Or go paint a theater set. Research from the MIT AgeLab has
highlighted this tiny subset of activities because it is an archetype
of positive volunteer work: physically active, group-oriented, and
almost invariably intergenerational. You don't need to rush to the
paint store, but consider volunteer opportunities that foster these
critical sets of values.

Treat volunteering as part of your retirement career. Never forget the lessons of Table 23. The younger people were inspired and
excited by the next twenty years, making big plans for their careers,
their lives, and their community. The older people weren't. They
acted as if their next twenty had less value, that they weren't worth
the effort to plan for, to optimize and make productive. It makes so
little sense. Older people have more experience and a greater ability to plan for the future. They have decades of learning on what
works and what doesn't, both in general and for themselves. Research shows that the years after sixty are some of the happiest and
most settled years of people's lives. The U-curve of happiness, as it
is called, shows that we are at our happiest in early and late life.[40] It
would be bad manners to mention them at a wedding, but all sorts
of pitfalls and challenges can await Sarah and Jay. The path forward
for Sarah's mother's law school roommate's husband is far clearer.
Later life is not without its very hard challenges, let's not gloss over

that, and the physical, cognitive, and emotional challenges of late life should not be underestimated, but we will all do better if we embrace the possibilities of the next twenty years. Treat them as a new, exciting phase of life, and consider volunteering as part of a larger portfolio of your next act. It can be the centerpiece, or it can be a sideline to work or learning or any other significant sets of activities. Make a plan, have goals, and treat the next twenty years as seriously and meticulously as you did the last twenty.

Chapter 5

The Last Acceptable "Ism"

THE MODEL EASES down the runway. She twirls and shimmies so the audience can get the full flavor of her flowing Chinese dress. The applause and exclamations from the audience are loud and enthusiastic, easily drowning out the tinny, cheap speakers that are gamely trying to pace the model's walk. Her partner follows steps behind. He's wearing a vest and cap and he's cradling a pipe, his outfit vaguely reminiscent of Paul Newman in *The Sting*, though the resemblance stops rather abruptly at the clothing. They are perhaps not the most graceful models I've ever seen, but to be fair, the room doesn't show them off all that well.

Thirty minutes earlier, the room had looked like a senior center, because that's what the Mei Ling Active Aging Centre in Singapore is, and it had been crowded with tables, lunch foods, and roughly seventy hungry, excited senior citizens. The catwalk, if you want to call it that, was little more than a narrow path that had been cleared through the tables, and the models for the show were either members or volunteers at the senior center ranging in age from sixty-five to nearly ninety. The improvised nature of the show did nothing to reduce the enthusiasm in the room, as every step and pirouette was greeted with cheering that felt more enthusiastic and genuine than anything you would see at New York Fashion Week.

The raucous audience notwithstanding, the show had an impromptu feel to it because this version was put together on barely a day's notice. It's a miniature version of a much larger show that was held just months before. The video of that show was playing in the background, largely for my benefit, but to the great enjoyment of everyone in the room nonetheless. That show, as well as today's activities, had been organized by the Lions Befrienders, a social organization in Singapore that runs dozens of active aging centers including Mei Ling, and it had drawn hundreds of spectators of all ages from across the city. Unlike today's obstacle course, the original event had professional production: a commercially sized stage, quality lighting, a sound system that was not tuned to someone's iPhone, and a full coterie of older models who followed a carefully choreographed route down the runway. It was intended to be fun for participants and audiences—and it was that—but the organizers and models were also making a statement: That even in fashion and modeling—a social fortress for the young and beautiful if there ever was one—older people can hold their own and carve their own path, one that is not bounded by outdated notions of what older people can and should do. I don't think Lions Befrienders has aspirations to challenge the Singaporean fashion industry, but it was sending out a clear message that the second half of life is as vigorous and creative, and beautiful, as the first.

The Lions Befrienders fashion show is not entirely unique—I've found a similar event at Fashion Week Minnesota and even happened upon a modeling agency in Tel Aviv that specializes exclusively in older models—but in Singapore, it is more than a one-off. It is a mirror of how Singaporeans in general and older Singaporeans in particular view the second half of life as a time of opportunity, freedom, and innovation. It's reflected in how Singaporeans talk about their lives and in how they respond to survey questions: Large percentages of older Singaporeans want to continue to work, make new friendships, learn new skills, and give back through volunteering. These aspirations give older Singaporeans a greater sense of possibility and autonomy: Two-thirds say that their age rarely or never stops them from doing the things they want to do, and 80 percent say they are rarely or never left out of things.[1] Roughly two-thirds of older Singaporeans see themselves as role models for aging, reflecting a positive spirit associated with old age that is lacking in many societies. And older Singaporeans are supported by the broader community. About 70 percent of older Singaporeans report that older people are well respected in society, and over 95 percent say that they have rarely or ever been the subject of age discrimination or poor treatment because of their age. Compare that to Germany, where 20 percent of older people report age discrimination, or the UK at 33 percent, or even Finland at 43 percent.

In part, the differences in perceived ageism reflect civil society's efforts to reduce ageism both in the workplace and in the broader community. Combating ageism isn't a priority, or even a consideration, for most in the US or the UK,[2] but it is in Singapore. Over the last decade, the Singaporean government has rolled out one initiative after another: public awareness campaigns, training programs, and even rule settings in support of a more age-inclusive society. Some of the actions are small, barely perceptible outside the halls of government, but others involve rethinking the roles of entire government agencies. Take, for instance, the Agency for Integrated Care (AIC). It started out modestly in 1992 as the Care Liaison Service, tasked with placing the elderly sick in nursing homes and other congregate care facilities. A decade later, it had rebranded itself as Integrated Care Services and taken on additional functions, but it was still largely focused on traditional health care services for the elderly.[3]

By 2018, Singapore was moving rapidly to the notion that a supportive aging environment should focus on helping people age healthfully rather than just having a well-treated sickly populace. The once again rebranded Agency for Integrated Care was at the center of this effort, tasked with the responsibility of implementing the "Healthy SG" plan. In 2023, as a core part of that strategy, the AIC launched a multifaceted anti-ageism campaign called "Break the Silver Ceiling." The campaign centered on public service messaging that ran on digital and social platforms, but the fun part was a series of pop-up events across Singapore. My favorite: a five-person, twenty-four-kilometer relay run across the city on a wildly circuitous route that if you laid it out on paper spelled "Boomer is OK," a play on the notorious OK boomer trope.[4] It was weird for sure, but also kind of wonderful that an agency which not so long ago specialized in efficiently allocating patients to nursing homes was now trying to win the public over with positive messaging around aging.

If there was no ageism or age discrimination in Singapore, the government wouldn't have to run campaigns or design wickedly convoluted racecourses, but even acknowledging that, the baseline for ageism in Singapore is much lower than in the West. Singaporean society, like many of the societies of East Asia, has been built on Confucian fundamentals. It may have been 2,500 years since

Confucious penned "Might we not say that filial piety and respect for elders constitute the root of Goodness," but those principles still permeate Singaporean culture. Deference to older people, and more importantly a respect for their knowledge and wisdom, runs deep in collectivist cultures like Singapore's, and that, as we shall shortly see, has an enormous impact on healthy aging.

———

If you have heard of Galicia, the small province in northwest Spain that sits like a cap on top of Portugal, you most likely know it in connection with the Camino de Santiago, or the Way of St. James in English, one of the three great pilgrimages of Christendom. Since at least the tenth century, pilgrims have been making their way over the mountains, mostly on foot but sometimes on donkeys, to the Cathedral of Santiago de Compostela, where tradition holds the remains of the Apostle James are buried.

Down the road from Santiago de Compostela is Ourense, which you might think of as the second city of Galicia. It has more modest claims to fame. The Ponte Vella is one of the oldest remaining usable Roman bridges in the world. Originally constructed in the first century during the reign of Emperor Augustus, the bridge is open today only to foot traffic, but its thick stone footings make it feel solid enough, two thousand years on, to hold a convoy of trucks. The bridge is not far from the thermal baths that are probably the city's biggest tourist attractions today.

But if you ask people in Ourense what sets them apart, they tend to eschew the tourist attractions and instead tout the extraordinary number of centenarians and older people in the town and the region. Galicia in general, and Ourense in particular, claims the largest concentrations of centenarians in all of Spain and Europe, and that fact is an enormous source of civic pride. Centenarians are more than just a point of curiosity for Ourense. They are seen as proof points of what makes Galicia special and, as a consequence, the centenarians of Galicia are treated as celebrities, and tales are swapped about their vigor. During my visit, several people urged me to visit Miss Esperanza, age 107, who still attends dances twice a week and is known to complain if her younger, think octogenarian, partners are insufficiently vigorous. I'd need to bring my A game, I was assured, if I wanted to keep up with Miss Esperanza. It's been a long time since I've had any game on the dance floor, let alone an A game, so I passed on that opportunity, but the admiring, almost reverential, way that everyone spoke about Miss Esperanza and her super-aged peers stuck with me.

The memories of my visit to Ourense came tumbling back when I was reading about strikingly similar experiences that the aging researcher Becca Levy had in Japan. As a Harvard graduate student, Levy earned a National Science Foundation fellowship to spend a semester in Japan trying to understand why people there lived so long. She almost immediately noticed that the Japanese viewed old age quite differently from Americans, as an important stage of life that should be enjoyed rather than feared.[5] Older people, she observed, were treated with respect, their wisdom serving as a building block of civil society rather than a burden, a cost on life's expense ledger. She was startled to find that centenarians and supercentenarians were honored as celebrities, trotted out on television shows alongside pop stars, comics, and models.

And it is not just centenarians. Every third Monday in September, the Japanese celebrate Keiro no Hi, translated roughly as "Respect for the Aged Day." To us, that might sound like the equivalent of "Grandparents Day," a not-quite-real holiday that is remembered by few and observed by even fewer. National Ice Cream Day without the sprinkles. But Keiro no Hi is serious business in Japan. It's a national holiday where many offices shut down, and the trains are crowded as workers return home to honor their parents, grandparents, and the elderly more generally. Programs celebrating the elderly are aired on national television. Restaurants offer free meals, and volunteers bring specially prepared bento boxes of food to the housebound elderly. In smaller villages, schoolchildren prepare special dances and songs for a "keiro kai" show, with attendees treated to lunch, tea, and sweets after the performance.[6]

I used to ask my father—mostly kidding—why there was a Mother's Day and a Father's Day but no "Kid's Day," and he would tell me—mostly seriously—that "every day is kid's day." In Japan, every day feels a bit like Respect for the Aged Day. It's a country in which the elderly are viewed as "wise sages" and considered to be at the top of the social pyramid. Where else can you have a ninety-one-year-old woman, Tetsuko Kuroyanagi, holding down the top interview show on television and not have people grousing about the fact that she should make way for the next generation (or the next three generations, in her case)?[7]

Levy came away from her fellowship profoundly impressed by the culture of aging in Japan and with a deep desire to better understand the impact of culture, attitude, and ageism on health. It's not an intuitive idea that broad cultural norms would affect blood pressure, increase the risk of diabetes, or accelerate cognitive decline, but Levy had an inkling that it could have an impact on physical health. After all, Japanese women, for example, are less likely to exhibit the hot flashes or other physical symptoms of menopause, an outgrowth Levy believed was a product of the more positive view of menopause and the aging process.[8] But her thought ran counter to the widespread assumption that afflictions from cardiovascular disease to dementia to diabetes were purely physical components of the aging process that operated independently of mental processes and beliefs.

In 2002, Levy began to crack open the medical consensus. Levy and her fellow researchers at Yale, where she now taught, had been studying a group of 660 people over the age of fifty who lived in the small town of Oxford, Ohio. The group was a perfect petri dish for Levy because they were part of a long-running study called the Ohio Longitudinal Study of Aging and Retirement, and she had access not only to health records dating back more than a generation but to participants' reactions to statements such as "as you get older, you get less useful." Sifting through the medical reports and the attitudinal data, Levy and her team made an astonishing discovery: The most important factor in determining the life expectancy and longevity of the test group—more important than functional health, income, education, and social background—was how they thought about and approached the idea of old age. The difference between those who had positive images of aging and those who did not amounted to almost eight years of life, even after holding constant for other factors. The life expectancy gap between the US and Japan at the time was only about 5.5 years, but if Levy was to be believed, much of that difference was attributable to the cultural script—how people in Japan assimilated widespread belief in the dignity and importance of aging, and people in the US inherited the opposite view that decline and dependency were the natural state of being old. It was an astonishing finding, one that has since been replicated in studies in countries as diverse as Australia, China, and Germany.

Over the years, Levy and other researchers have demonstrated that there are multiple pathways for ageism—or lack thereof—to influence our health, with an astonishing range of impact across our physical systems. People with positive images of aging recover faster from injury, and older adults primed with optimistic images of aging evidence improved memory. People with positive ideas about aging even hear and walk better than those with negative concepts around the second half of life.[9]

Ageism also has a direct and significant impact on the American health system. According to another study, this one in 2022, again led by the prolific Dr. Levy, $63 billion in costs—roughly one in every seven dollars spent on health care for older Americans—is traceable to the impact of ageism by driving up the incidence of eight of the ten most costly medical conditions (the other two are neonatal conditions), including cardiovascular disease, diabetes, mental disorders, and chronic respiratory disease.[10] To put this in perspective, the annual cost of ageism in America outweighs the estimated impact of its obesity crisis. Even a modest 10 percent reduction in ageism-related cases would decrease the number of cases requiring treatment by 1.7 million a year, resulting in billions of dollars in savings and untold human costs averted. It's a strong indictment of an ageist culture, and reflects the costs imposed not just on individuals, but on society as a whole.

Ageism takes many forms, with direct discrimination against older people in the workplace and in the health care system being among the most open and notorious. But rather astonishingly, the most destructive and costly aspect of ageism, studies have found, is not direct discrimination, nor negative age stereotypes held by younger people, but rather negative self-perceptions of aging adopted by older people themselves. Over the course of a lifetime, older people have been conditioned to think of themselves as less useful, more forgetful, and less worthy of respect—with the result that older people are less inclined to seek social connection and support and invest less in taking good care of themselves. To quote Pogo Possum from the comic strip *Pogo*: "We have met the enemy and he is us."

Given the relationship between our own self-perception and health, it is not terribly surprising to learn that ageism can also have a large impact on cognitive functions. In 2023, Levy and her colleagues published the results of a multi-year study of thousands of older adults suffering from Mild Cognitive Impairment (MCI), a category of mental decline just below dementia.[11] MCI can have a significant impact on functioning by itself, and can also be a stepping stone to dementia, but not for everyone. Some older adults recover normal functioning—and the Yale team found that attitudes about aging were one of the most significant markers of whether someone would recover or not. In fact, older adults were 30 percent more likely to regain normal cognitive function if they had a positive view of aging. The research team also found that those with positive attitudes and beliefs about aging were likely to recover up to two years earlier than those with negative beliefs. The data lays bare how older adults, especially in Western countries, frequently internalize society's negative views of aging—with direct and often dramatic cost to their own health and mental functioning.

It is perhaps not intuitively obvious why having poor conceptions of aging translates so dramatically to poorer health. While researchers are quite clear that ageist concepts have a dramatic impact on health and life expectancy, the mechanisms for that impact have been perceived as more ambiguous. But there is now an emerging consensus that ageist conceptions have at least two distinct ways of impacting health and longevity. If you associate aging with decline, physical infirmity, and a bumpy glide path toward death, then getting old is going to be depressing and stressful, and both mental health challenges and elevated stress levels—and the resulting increases in inflammation and cortisol levels—are highly correlated with poor health.

At the same time, if you are depressed about getting old, you may very well believe that self-improvement is futile and therefore forego opportunities to improve your health. Ageism increases risky health behaviors, such as eating an unhealthy diet, drinking excessively, or smoking. If you think that you are in a rapid slide toward the end, the evidence shows, you're more likely to add bacon to that double cheeseburger, reach for that fourth drink, or skip that unpleasant colonoscopy than you would if you thought you still had good years to live. In the same vein, if you associate aging with memory loss and poor cognitive health, the idea of engaging in learning, for instance, is also going to be perceived as a waste of time. Ultimately, the thinking goes, if you think getting old inevitably means being frail and mentally infirm, you're going to get your wish.

In places like the US and the UK, we are conditioned to associate aging with cognitive decline and failing memory. I vividly recall my own mother decrying her lack of recall, telling me that "getting old is not for the faint of heart." But we forget things when we are young, middle-aged, and old, and it is only when we are older that we associate temporary forgetfulness with our stage of life. Scientists still have much to learn about neuroplasticity, but we know that some forms of memory—such as episodic memory—do decline with age, while other forms of memory—such as procedural memory and semantic memory—either stay the same as we age or even improve. There is a lot of complexity around aging and memory, but the evidence is increasingly showing that it is not a one-way street. In China, where elders are treated with great respect, research has shown that older Chinese test similarly to their grandchildren in terms of the effectiveness of memory.[12]

The anti-ageism crusader Ashton Applewhite has described America as "grotesquely youth-centric."[13] I'm not sure that I would go quite that far. Older Americans are surely poorly treated in our culture, but they are well-treated when it comes to the division of our national financial and political resources. I have friends in Gen Z who with some cause think the deck is stacked against their generation, not older ones, though I don't see many offering to change places with me. We can acknowledge legitimate questions about the distribution of resources and authority, but that doesn't obscure the fact that we generally view older age as something between an embarrassment and a moral failing, a time of life to be avoided or at least lied about as long as you can get away with it. At best, we have an ambivalent relationship with the idea of aging. The public pride in the doubling of life expectancy over the last century and a half, truly one of the great achievements of modern society, is substantially leavened by the fact that we associate aging with weakness, decline, and selfishness.

Some Western commentators have an answer to that question. In Anthony Trollope's 1882 novel *The Fixed Period*, the fictional island nation of Britannula, located near New Zealand, solves the problem of aging with mandatory euthanasia at age sixty-eight. That seems gentle, positively balanced, compared to the dystopian movie *Logan's Run*. In the 1976 cult classic, the societies of the twenty-third century have chosen to deal with the challenges of rising population and finite resources by sending everyone on their thirtieth birthday to Carousel, described as a rite of renewal but in reality an execution. Inevitably, the plot revolves around one of the Sandmen—charged with ensuring that no one escapes Carousel—having a convenient late-life conversion on the ethics of the matter and trying to escape. At least we can view *The Fixed Period* and *Logan's Run* as satire and social commentary. It's much harder to do that with seriously offered commentary, such as multiple comments from Texas Lieutenant Governor Dan Patrick during the COVID-19 pandemic that older people should be willing to sacrifice themselves so that the economy could remain fully open.[14] I don't doubt that many older people would be willing to sacrifice themselves to save the lives of their progeny, but fewer, it seemed, were eager to do so for the right to shop at Costco.

It's often assumed that the "collectivist" societies of East Asia and Latin America—those built on strong family and community cultures—are less ageist than the individualistic societies of the West. It makes sense. One of the strongest predictors of ageism, as is often said of other "isms" as well, is lack of exposure to viable role models. Having close contact with older people tends to reduce intergenerational hostility. Modernity has reduced the ubiquity of the multigenerational family in places like Japan and Korea, but it remains far more visible and viable as a building block of society there than in the West, and elders continue to play a much more central role in family and community life.

But for years, it remained just an assumption—a logical one but still an assumption—that ageism was relatively high in the individualistic and increasingly accusatory societies of the West and relatively low in the collectivist cultures of East Asia, Latin America, and Africa. There were polls, of course, and studies here or there, but you couldn't take anything definitive away from it: The datasets were different, the questions asked of respondents varied from place to place, and researchers were a little bit at cross purposes. Some were interested, for instance, in discrimination in the workplace, while others focused on how self-perception was influenced by media portrayal of older people. It was all a bit of a mess for that relatively small group of people who wanted to compare ageism across nations and cultures.

All of that has now changed, in substantial part thanks to Bill Chopik, an associate professor of psychology and head of the Close Relationships Lab at Michigan State University. Chopik is a relative rarity in academia: He's young—in his late thirties now—and principally studies ageism and older people. When I ask him how he got interested in aging issues, he credits his close relationship with his grandparents, which is almost always the answer you get. But there must not be enough grandparents to go around, because there is a large deficit in those who take care of, create products for, and research the needs of older people. Take gerontology, for example. Despite the rapid increase in the population over sixty-five, the number of gerontologists in the US has steadily declined over the years. The American Geriatrics Society estimates that an average gerontologist can take care of seven hundred patients, but the ratio of gerontologists to geriatric patients in the US is closer to one to ten thousand.[15] It's a reflection of how the medical profession, and society, values older people.

The same is true in academia. In recent years, American universities have encouraged and supported the expansion of scholarship of a vast range of issues related to discrimination based on race, gender, sexual orientation, and country of origin, for instance, while research focused on ageism and age has waned. It's not a competition—age would lose out anyway if it were—but it says something about a country in which one of the fastest-growing parts of the population is badly underserved by marketers, academia, and medical professionals alike.

But not Chopik, who has built his academic career around studying the impact of ageism, both in the US and comparatively around the world. One of the issues that has always motivated him has been to understand the differences in attitudes on aging between cultures, and how to study that on more than an anecdotal basis. In 2020, he unearthed a dataset of over nine hundred thousand adults from sixty-four countries that included an entire battery of questions that explored implicit and explicit biases on age. Some of the questions tried to get at ageism with simple measures of explicit bias: Rate on a scale of one to five how you feel about older people, for instance. Other parts of the dataset were a little more complex. Respondents were asked to match pictures of younger people and older people with positive qualities; researchers measured how long it took to make a match and whether it took longer (it usually did) to associate positive qualities with the pictures of the older people than with the photos of the younger people. The gap between the two is considered a measure of ageism.

But perhaps the most interesting question focused on "how old do you feel?" For younger people, it's kind of a strange question. An eighteen-year-old almost always feels like an eighteen-year-old. Same for the thirty-five-year-old. But as you get toward older ages, forty-five, fifty, sixty, a certain amount of cognitive dissonance sets in because being old is associated with ill health and decline, and people connect any good health or vigor with younger ages. It's banal now to say that you feel much younger than your actual age—I've said many times at age sixty that I don't feel older than fifty, and sometimes I slip it down to forty-five if I'm feeling particularly frisky, without even thinking that it is an implicit and negative referendum on what I think sixty should feel like. It's not a perfect measure of ageism, of course; a lot of things go into these types of statements, but it's revealing nonetheless. It turns out that in many places in the West, like the UK and Switzerland, there are very large gaps for older people between actual age and perceived age. Older people in Korea, Singapore, and Taiwan, on the other hand, register virtually no difference. In Chopik's analysis, collectivist, family-oriented countries like Korea, Japan, and Singapore consistently score on the positive end of ageism, and more individualistic countries like the US, the UK, Canada, and Australia skew steeply toward the very bottom of the rankings.

Other researchers have reached similar conclusions, though with very different methodologies. For instance, Reuben Ng, a scholar at the National University of Singapore, has tried to get at the issue of comparative ageism by analyzing a dataset of some twenty-eight million articles across twenty countries. Intriguingly, he found that it is the relative masculinity of the society that would be determinative of ageism.[16] More masculine societies that tend to "emphasize competition and favor the strong and successful may systematically frame elders as weak, leading to the development of ageism at the societal level." It's a different take on the issue but it nets out at the same place, with male-dominated societies such as the UK, the US, and Canada at the top of the ageism list.

I'm glad to have the certainty of quantitative data, but it's just confirmatory of things we see in everyday life. In the week that I was working on this chapter in June 2024, the top-grossing movie in Singapore was *How to Make Millions Before Grandma Dies*, a complex but ultimately heartwarming story that follows an aimless (and broke) young man named M as he volunteers to take care of his maternal grandmother who is struggling with stage 4 cancer.[17] The movie follows M as he navigates his complicated, multigenerational Thai-Chinese household and his hero's journey from being motivated by avarice toward his grandmother's will to finding true appreciation for family, responsibility, and love. The top-grossing movie in the US and the UK that same week was *Bad Boys: Ride or Die*. It's an interesting comparison because you can make the argument that *Bad Boys* is an anti-ageist movie, as the heroes of the movie—if you are willing to define heroism as a cheerful predilection for violence and rule-breaking—are two graying men in their late fifties. This is how Hollywood is beginning to grapple with the changing demographics of their audience: by insisting that the Will Smith of 2024 is not any different than the Will Smith of 1995, when the first *Bad Boys* came out. It's better, I suppose, than substituting in a younger actor, a la James Bond, but we're left with the message that successful aging is acting exactly as you did thirty years before. I don't want to make too much of the differences—it's just one movie after all, and the latest *Bad Boys* grossed $100 million outside the

US—but it is difficult to ignore the very different perspectives on aging and intergenerational relationships in the competing films.

Ageism is a drag on health in many places in the US, but it is not evenly distributed. Chopik also studied comparative ageism on a state-by-state basis and found that ageism was highest in the snowbird states like Florida and Arizona where older people gather in large numbers. It tracks, Chopik told me, generational resentments around the division of resources, and it also reflects the strong self-segregation of society in those places. Instead of bringing the generations together to build connections and common ground, transplants end up in walled communities populated only by people of their own age. It's the worst of all possible worlds. Lots of people from all generations, and none of them knowing one another. Ageism in the US is often referred to as the last socially acceptable "ism," and it appears to be particularly acceptable in the Sunbelt, much to the detriment of society in general and older people in particular.

—

I had started the Asian leg of my travels in Seoul in March, when daytime temperatures hovered in the fifties and the evenings had a delightful nip to them. By the time I reached Singapore a month later, the thermometer had turned against me, topping ninety degrees every day. And if you add in the humidity to get one of those "feels like" temperatures, as the meteorologists sometimes do, it registered at about two degrees short of heatstroke. So when I see Snow City, which promises ice slides and the world's coldest bumper car arena, it takes all my willpower to bypass those delights and ignore the promised enchantments of Professor Crackitt's Light Fantastic Mirror Maze as well.

I'm not at the Singapore Science Centre for any of that. I'm here to visit an exhibit titled "Dialogue with Time—Embracing Aging." I make it past Snow City, skip past the good professor, and arrive at the exhibit, where I am greeted by Siva. She's seventy-three and has been a docent since the exhibit opened eight years before. Her job is to walk me through a series of displays and presentations that have two interlocking purposes: building empathy for the challenges of aging and reframing the years past sixty-five not as years of decline, but as a time of productivity, purpose, and social contribution. It's the question that the Science Centre plasters in front of the exhibit: "How can society and the way we live our lives be shaped to maximize the opportunities of longevity?" It's not a question that the schoolchildren who make up the bulk of the visitors to the exhibit typically think about, and initiating dialogue around this at an early stage of life is right out of the Singaporean playbook: developing a cultural consensus that views the second half of life as just as important and productive as the first.

Siva herself is a good example. Born in Malaysia, she immigrated to Singapore with her husband and forged a successful career at the Ministry of Health. Since retiring, she has found renewed purpose in working at the Science Centre and tells me, as she tells the schoolchildren, that she continues to learn and grow. She illustrates this with a story of overcoming her fear of snorkeling. It doesn't particularly impress me—snorkeling is easy, bypassing Snow City is hard—but the message is clear: Learning, personal growth, and being a little daring are not values unique to the young. They are attributes of the curious mind and heart which can be present (or missing) at any age.

Empathy is a central element of Dialogue with Time. Siva walks me through a series of tests to show how older people might experience physical challenges. Some I handle easily: Strapping five-pound weights to each leg and climbing stairs presents no obstacles, though Siva rather unkindly deflates my ego a bit when she points out that the typical customer here is an eleven-year-old child. Some prove much more difficult, at least for me. I press my hand through a cylinder and grasp a key with the simple goal of inserting it into a lock. Not a great chore, similar to something I have done virtually every day of my life, but Siva flicks a switch, and the cylinder starts to shake, simulating the tremors that affect some older people. My hand shudders violently, far worse than if I've had too much to drink, and I fail spectacularly at getting the key to fit into the lock. It's not the only test that I fail. Siva invites me over to a table to play video games, but before I am allowed to play, my fingers are wrapped to replicate some of the sensory challenges associated with aging. With that handicap, I'm all thumbs and quickly lose. Other machines simulate macular degeneration and the challenge of filling a pill caddy when instructions come too fast. After my multiple failures, I'm rather too pleased with myself that I can master the pill caddy game so readily, and Siva again deflates me, unnecessarily really, reminding me of the core customers at the exhibit. It did occur to me that I might have gotten better treatment in Snow City, but overall, the whole experience leaves me both sympathetic to the challenges of aging and a little worried about how soon some of these challenges might come at me.

But the fundamental point of the Science Centre is not to scare children (and sixty-one-year-olds) about their future. Most of the exhibits feature older Singaporeans achieving great things. I'm ushered into a curtained booth, and a holographic picture of Ajit Singh Gill pops up in front of me. Gill is a storied athlete in Singaporean history. He represented the country at the 1956 Melbourne Olympics, the first Olympic Games in which Singapore participated as a separate country, and he later competed internationally as both a cricketer (he was saddled with the nickname of the "Big-hitting Sikh") and as a runner. In his video, he tells me with a touch of pride how he converted later in life to race walking, winning a gold medal at the ASEAN senior games held that year in Singapore. You can't watch the video and not be impressed with Ajit Singh's energy, strength, and vitality, though it leaves me with a touch of sadness when I discover the next day that he passed away at age ninety-five just weeks before my visit to Singapore.

The exhibit also tests expectations of what the second half of life should be. Siva shows me a deck of pictures and asks which one best reflects my conception of happiness in retirement. They are all upbeat photos, but older people like me tend to gravitate toward active scenes—travel or work, typically—while the younger visitors prefer the picture of a man relaxing in a beach chair in a flower-strewn meadow. It looks lovely, I have to admit, but it won't appeal to anyone who conceives of the years past sixty as a period of activity, purpose, and social contribution. But it does show that even in Singapore, traditional constructs that associate retirement with idleness start early and are deeply enmeshed in the culture.

As a final stop, Siva ushers me into a small theater and invites me to take a quiz about the super-aged society that Singapore will soon be. I'm a little nervous because my track record on these types of quizzes is not very good, despite my self-proclaimed expertise on healthy aging. Earlier in the year, I had volunteered to take a geography quiz, authored by our eight-year-old neighbor, Milo. I had assumed it would be a breeze, but it proved shockingly hard (go ahead, you tell me what country touches both the equator and the Tropic of Capricorn). But on the question of what country has the world's longest life expectancy, I confidently answer Japan. Milo draws a red slash through my answer, telling me that the correct answer is Monaco, and my appeal that "countries" with populations under forty thousand don't really count is rejected by the court of second grade. I do a little better in the Science Centre, but again I'm caught off guard by the fact that Singapore is already home to 1,400 centenarians, a doubling from just ten years ago, and, Milo, please take note—a whole lot more than in Monaco. For the school kids of Singapore, there is a clear message: The Singapore of the future will look very different from the one that they know now, and that Singapore is preparing for a world in which older adults play a far more significant role in everyday life.

———

Lots of industries have contributed to our ageist cultures—media, technology, and entertainment all spring to mind—but if you ask me what industries have done the most to elevate the cult of the young, I would probably answer beauty and fashion. For decades, both industries, often in tandem, have built a multibillion-dollar business around the idea that everyone, but especially older women, should seek to look young, often in expensive and fundamentally unattainable ways. Products are advertised as "anti-aging" as if there is something inherently unattractive in aging; Dior went so far in 2017 as to name twenty-five-year-old Cara Delevingne as the face of its anti-aging skincare line Capture Youth, a move that was met with a certain amount of skepticism that the forty-, fifty-, and sixty-year-old women who were the targets of the campaign should aspire to look like an unblemished model half their age. As the demographic for beauty products has aged, the industry has gotten a little cagier about language—dropping terms like "anti-aging"—but the underlying goal of persuading older people to feel bad that they don't look like younger people remains an underlying industry ethic.

You might be tempted to view this as a universal trait, and certainly there are plenty of rail-thin fashion models in Tokyo and Milan, but in many of these places, the youth-oriented slant is alleviated by a much larger presence for older people and a sense that norms of beauty mature as we age. Duck into any newsstand in Seoul and peruse the fashion magazines. Instead of the obsession with youth, you will see a far more demographically accurate depiction of society. Young people, old people, and families grace the magazines, reflecting the fact that older adults can be seen and heard in Korean society—and explaining why so many older people can feel comfortable expressing themselves through fashion.

Some of those pictures in the newsstand may very well come from Kim Donghyun. I may not be cool myself, but I sometimes can recognize it in others, and Kim is cool, or "mut," as he translates from Korean. When I meet him at his cramped studio perched on the rooftop of an apartment block in western Seoul, he is dressed in that casual way that says, "I've spent a lot of time, and maybe money, trying to look casual." His hard-rimmed black glasses frame alert eyes, which you would expect from someone who has forged his reputation as a street photographer.

I'd place Kim in his early thirties, which is rather young for having made himself the chronicler of older fashionistas around

Seoul—men and women in their sixties, seventies, eighties, and even nineties who have that mut from a combination of dressing fashionably and being comfortable in their own skin. His studio sprouts photos of older Koreans dressed in everything from biker chic to tie-dye retro to banker pinstripe—and they also grace the pages of some of the most influential fashion magazines in the country, including *Vogue Korea*. Among his favorite spreads is that of his grandmother. He pages through *Vogue* to show me a picture of her decked out in a bold purple-on-white jacket with a matching white-on-purple scarf. The next photo zooms in on her aging hands, centered on the gold wedding band that never comes off even fifteen years after the death of Kim's grandfather. They are captivating photos, reflecting both the passion that Kim brings to his work and the timeless beauty of his subjects.

Kim didn't start off to be a photographer of older adults; in fact, as a young fashion student it never really occurred to him that older adults could have their own sense of style. But he chose the nearby Dongmyo Flea Market, a sprawling outdoor venue known for both low prices and vintage clothing, as a background for his early street photographer efforts. To his surprise, he found the market had become a cultural hub for older adults, a playground for those who appreciated fashion and had developed their own personal look over the course of decades. He admired these older fashionistas, as he calls them, and the fact that they had the courage to pursue their own style and unique ways of expressing their individuality. It led him to the epiphany that "style has no age."[18]

It sometimes feels like ageism is so deeply ingrained in American and Western cultures that it is eternal, a fundamental part of who we are. But that's not quite true. It wasn't so long ago that age played a much less significant role in our identity—many people didn't even know how old they were well into the nineteenth century—and there are important, though limited, reevaluations already happening. Even in the fashion industry, fingered just a couple pages ago as a prime offender on ageism, some change is afoot. At Fashion Week Paris in 2024, older models (defined as older than thirty-five) abounded. Roughly three-quarters of the top twenty runway shows in both Paris and Milan featured at least one older model. At the shows held by the Vetements and Schiaparelli fashion houses, the figure was closer to one-fifth of all models cast,[19] and the Batsheva fashion house topped them all by using only models over the age of forty for its New York show earlier in the year.[20] The Hispanitas fashion brand in Spain has similarly made older models the centerpiece of their new campaigns. And L'Oréal, the French beauty company, has put its mark on the space by launching the L'Oréal for All Generations efforts, which focuses on building the intergenerational workforce, supporting training and employability across the entire career and helping older workers as they transition to retirement or their next act. L'Oréal is, in fact, one of the relatively few companies, in beauty or elsewhere, that have identified age diversity as a central element of their overall diversity and inclusion efforts.

This all reflects, one might speculate, the changing economics of fashion and clothing, where an increasingly large percentage of customers are over fifty and sixty, and the dawning realization that it makes good business sense to show older customers how they can look not only attractive but also authentic. I don't want to get too moony over the fact that not all fashion models are being pushed off the dock at the ripe old age of thirty anymore, but money does have a way of subverting cultural norms.

Market conditions may be slowly driving commerce in the right direction, but ageism still has its long tentacles in our culture. To combat this, some countries have even launched public relations campaigns to counter ageism. The UK has Age Without Limits; Australia has EveryAGE Counts. These are worthy efforts, no doubt, though it is still uncomfortably common to see someone run down on social media because they are old or casually dismissed because they are boomers.[21] Whatever progress there is, we still have a long way to go.

Hiro and I arrive early for our appointment in a small, mixed-use neighborhood in north central Tokyo. Most of the buildings are low-slung, two to three stories at most, and overshadowed by the power and phone lines that frame every street like a modern art project. Tokyo is an incredibly tidy city—there aren't even any public waste cans since everyone buses their own trash—so the double helices of tangled power lines seem jarringly out of place. It's a concession to environmental vulnerability in Japan. Buried power lines are impossible to reach after an earthquake, so the poor aesthetics are viewed as an acceptable cost of emergency response.

Power lines aren't the only things that loom over the neighborhood. Towering over the squat buildings is an imposing twenty-seven-story structure, the home of the Yamano Beauty School. It required special dispensation to build such a tall building in an otherwise uniformly flat neighborhood (I can only imagine the litigation that would ensue in the United States), but the school is a source of civic pride in the area, and a deal was quickly struck to allow them to circumvent the zoning code. It's strange for me as an American to think of a beauty school as an important cultural institution—I would think of it as a trade school if I thought of it at all—but Yamano has cultural currency far beyond the two thousand or so students who attend the beauty school and its sister beauty college. Yamano, now almost a century old, was an early pioneer of a unique Japanese philosophy of aging: That beauty is a reflection in part of outer beauty (hair, makeup, and dress) but also the beauty of physical health, mental health, and social worth. It nourishes the view that older people—and let's be specific that we are talking mostly older women—can be beautiful on their own terms as they age and project their true selves outward through their evolving physical appearance.

It's not merely lip service. In addition to taking classes in makeup, coloring, and hair curling, students at Yamano are tutored in psychology, social engagement, and gerontology through a unique partnership with the Leonard Davis School of Gerontology at the University of Southern California. Students also take frequent field trips to nursing homes, senior centers, and other congregate facilities to offer beauty services to older adults. In total, it reflects at once a revolutionary and intrinsically Japanese view of helping people age gracefully, which is why both founders of the school—Aiko and Jiichi Yamano, as well as their eldest son, Mike, who ran the company after their death—have been awarded medals of service by the emperors of Japan.

After we finish our visit at Yamano, Hiro and I share a laugh at how out of place we must have looked. I'm always a bit rumpled, and three weeks on the road have done my clothes and me no favors. And even if I were at the top of my game, which I rarely am, I would pale in comparison to our hosts. Jane Yamano is beautifully dressed and arranged, even I can tell that. And her husband, Stan, who serves as a senior advisor in the company, is immaculately tailored, his suit decorated with a tie from the British clothier Thomas Pink that is not quite blue and not quite emerald but something delightfully in between. Yet I don't feel self-conscious at Yamano. The school celebrates the idea that you can look good at your own pace and in your own style, and that's more important than competing to look as youthful as possible. It's why Yamano can recognize norms of beauty that are universal but also help older adults feel that they are still beautiful as they age. It's a critical concept in an aging society where value and sense of worth are central to the goals of aging healthfully.

Revolutionary thinking comes naturally at Yamano. The school was founded in 1934 by Aiko Yamano, who as a woman, and a young one at that, had an unusual profile for a company founder. Born in 1909, Aiko began working in the beauty industry in 1925, largely as a product of circumstances. At the time, Tokyo was still struggling to recover from the devastating effects of the Great Kanto Earthquake of 1923, which killed an estimated 142,000 people and leveled vast swaths of the town. Jane Yamano, who is now the third generation of the family to run the company, told me that demand for beauty services often spikes in the wake of natural disasters as people try to find some respite and normalcy in life, and so it was in the aftermath of the Kanto earthquake. Aiko Yamano saw an opportunity and began opening up beauty shops around Tokyo. Nine years later, seeing increased competition in the beauty industry and the hundreds of young women aspiring to enter the field, she pivoted and opened up the first (and now the largest) beauty school in the country.

From the beginning, Yamano, both the school and the person, attached a broader meaning to the idea of beauty. Aiko articulated a new philosophy of beauty, which she dubbed Bido, roughly meaning "the road of beauty," and she described five elements of this philosophy: hair, face, dress, physical health, and mental health. None by themselves would amount to beauty. Only all five elements, joined together, would amount to true beauty, and students were taught to care for all aspects of the person. It's a philosophy that has guided the Yamano schools ever since, influencing both industry and culture for nearly a century.

Beauty standards and cultural norms are particularly important to healthy aging because women not only live longer than men, but also live more years (and a higher percentage of years) in poor health. It's sometimes called the "gender and age paradox," and it can produce startling numbers: In the US, as of 2019, just before the COVID-19 pandemic, life expectancy at birth for women was 4.5 years longer than for men, but women live 13.8 years in poor health compared to only 11.1 for men.[22] The existence of a gap in healthy aging and healthy longevity exists across the world but tends to be larger in high-income countries. Women's disadvantage in healthy aging stems from greater vulnerability to a wide variety of syndromes but is most acute around mental health. Women worldwide are more susceptible to depressive disorders and anxiety disorders, and both play a substantial role in the healthy aging disparity, especially in those high-income countries.[23] Many factors influence these outcomes, including greater economic and physical vulnerability for women. Research on healthy aging gaps between women and men is relatively primitive at this stage, but gendered ageism and reduced sense of self-worth no doubt play a critical role in the women's health disparities, at least in the US. The fact that Yamano has for more than a century reset cultural norms to help women is a key reason that it holds such an honored place in Tokyo and Japan.

In many ways, it is not surprising that the Yamano Beauty School has pushed cultural norms since the spirit of innovation is etched deeply into its DNA. In the 1930s, when the Japanese military started confiscating all metal right down to hair pins for the war effort, Aiko Yamano responded by inventing a new braided look for women, requiring no hair pins, that became the fashion of the day and for decades after. Her husband, Jiichi, also played a significant role in the evolution of the Yamano business. He created the first industry standards for beauty schools and was also the first to bring a perm machine to Japan, a somewhat meaningless accomplishment to a writer who transitioned from balding to bald many years ago, but undoubtedly more significant to the millions of Japanese women who flocked to try it. The first machine still sits in the family museum, looking like a metal jellyfish with a rounded top and dangling metal strings. It appears decidedly uncomfortable, but it was an instant hit with salons and customers across the country.

Aiko was an innovator not only in business but also in her personal life. After finding financial success with her salons and the beauty school, she decided her next challenge would be to build a family. Not content to follow traditional social patterns, she sought out matchmakers to help her find a husband. Eventually judging Jiichi to be a suitable match, she carefully negotiated with him the terms of their marriage, the details of which are memorialized in writing at the Yamano family museum. Rather rare for the time, and even now for that matter, Jiichi agreed to take on the Yamano name since it had economic currency, and they both consented to a ten-year initial run to the marriage, subject to renewal if mutually agreeable. The contract also specified terms around business and children; the couple would establish a new beauty shop every time Aiko bore a child (which she did six times). It seems astonishingly bloodless, but it worked for them, as they renewed the contract every nine or ten years until their death. But more importantly for my purposes, the episode reveals Aiko for what she was: unafraid to buck convention, willing to push social norms, and kind of a badass to boot.

Aiko passed away in 1995 at the age of eighty-six. It is, in any era, a good, long life, but in fact it is now two years short of the average life expectancy and four years short of the median lifespan of Japanese women, which is now almost exactly ninety.[24] While Japanese women are not quite to the lifespans of Prester John's happy kingdom, they are getting surprisingly close and will only get closer in the future.

There are many factors that go into the long, healthy life of Japanese women, but one of them is surely that women in old age are treated with great respect. Women in Japan, research has shown, in turn view old age as a particularly good time of life because of their favorable position in society—the fact that they may now have been relieved of difficult childcare responsibilities, allowing for more time and disposable income to pursue personal passions.[25] It's good to be old in Japan, a view that unfortunately you don't hear often in the US, the UK, or any other country that has bought into ageist norms of the twentieth and the twenty-first centuries.

Three Tips for Healthy Aging

We all have a stake in ageism as someday, we can hope, we're going to be old. You might expect older people to be vigorous opponents

of ageism—just as you might expect people of color to be most vigi-
lant on racism, women on sexism, and disabled people on ableism—
but it doesn't really work that way. We have a lifetime of absorbing
ageist assumptions, and it shows. But all of us can push back on
ageism for our own benefit and the benefit of society.

The question for us is: Do we associate aging with a new chapter of life or with a narrative of decay and decline? At Table 23, the
weight of society's ageism was on display. It was reflected in reduced
expectations for life and how we talked about the later years. Normal forgetfulness was chalked up to "senior moments," and aches
and diseases of advancing years were offered up as conversational
trophies. I don't want to leave you with the impression that all we
did at dinner was complain about aging—we complained about
politics as well—but the real shame was not in the precise details of
the conversation, but that we were doing it to ourselves. The good
news of doing it to yourself, however, is that it makes it that much
more straightforward to change the script.

Remodel your own language. On the surface, ageist language
seems, as Douglas Adams described Earth in *The Hitchhiker's Guide
to the Galaxy*, "mostly harmless." Who among us hasn't used phrases
like "you can't teach an old dog new tricks" or chalked up a moment
of forgetfulness to advancing age? But let's consider the cumulative impact. Language like this is often inaccurate, and not just in
semantic ways. You can teach old dogs (and humans) new tricks,
and while some aspects of learning, like processing speeds, decline
with age, other elements, like social learning, either don't decline
or may even improve with age. And while short-term memory
may slowly decline with age, it is hardly the case that losing things

or neglecting tasks are events uniquely associated with old age, as my frequent complaints to Nate can attest. This type of language paints a picture of old age as a period of decline and decrepitude, and while you might think of that as mostly harmless, it cumulatively reinforces unhealthy stereotypes. Simply remodeling your own language can help you think more positively about your own aging.

Own your age. I don't lie about my age, but I do often think (and say) that I feel younger than my actual age. No thanks to my three Diet Dr Pepper a day habit, I'm still in good health and in pretty good shape and can from time to time be heard saying "I don't feel sixty" or "I still feel forty." There is nothing wrong with feeling good—I wish the same for you—but implicitly we are saying that people at the age of sixty are likely unhealthy and entering a period of decline and diminishment. I'm not sure that I would select everyone at Table 23 first for our pickup basketball game, though I could do worse. Older age is a time of greater heterogeneity with respect to health and well-being, and there are plenty in my age cohort who are just as healthy and vigorous, or more, as I am. Let's rid ourselves of that assumption of what sixty or seventy or eighty looks like.

Invest in intergenerational relationships. Unfamiliarity is the handmaiden of ageism. Lack of contact between generations, not having positive older role models, is a fundamental source of ageist assumptions, and it is particularly virulent in the West in general and in places where young people feel displaced by older people. It's an unhealthy situation leading to bad results for older people today and younger people tomorrow. The best remedy for this is exploring intergenerational opportunities, whether at work, in your family, or more broadly in your community. I'm not saying that I am brave enough to swap seats with someone at Table 8, but breaking down barriers and building intergenerational relationships is a key strategy to combating ageism. It goes against decades of cultural segregation—but it is possible and necessary in a rapidly aging country and world.

Chapter 6

Wrinkles in Time

Building the Social Superhighway

THE BEST PHOTO I ever took, entirely by accident, was of a brilliant orange sunset over Presidio, its dusty main street and worn church bathed in a Sunkist glow that I would not have believed could be found in nature, but for this photo. If I had taken the shot five minutes later, the moment would have passed and the Presidio memorialized on my phone would have looked different, more average, more like every other rural community of the American Southwest.

I suspect, and am saddened at the thought, that Presidio's moment of good health will also pass, just like that reverential sunset, and be supplanted by life expectancy figures more typical of poor counties in the United States. Communities like Presidio tend not to survive the forces of social entropy. Roseto, a town in Pennsylvania once famous for its close social ties and provocatively good health, is now just another dot in the cancer cluster that runs from Allentown to Scranton.[1] And it's not just the United States. Places like Okinawa and the Nicoya Peninsula in Costa Rica, chronicled in the Blue Zones as places of low stress and healthy foods, are bending before the forces of technology, fast-food marketing, and social isolation.

Still, for the moment, Presidio seems to survive outside of time. The stores along O'Reilly Street, Presidio's main drag, are of a different era. Nieto's Department Store, which has been an anchor of O'Reilly Street since 1913, offers the same rough inventory as it has for a century. That is to say, it sells just about everything you might need, from clothing to washing machines, though now you can even have your packages delivered there, a nod to the encroaching presence of Amazon. The one newcomer is Pour-Over-Coffee, a softly lit, marbled café that would not look out of place in Houston or Dallas. It's owned by Sharon Hernandez, who in many ways is an unwilling stand-in for the pressures that places like Presidio face. You can see it on the streets of Presidio. Plenty of old people, a testament to the longevity of the area, but also a reflection of the fact that many younger people leave the town behind, pulled away by better jobs in the oil fields of Midland or by the charms of the big city. The latter was the case for Hernandez, who left for college in Dallas without an intention to return, despite the contrary wishes of her family. But seventeen years later, half of her life, the COVID-19 pandemic brought her back to her childhood bedroom, Backstreet Boys posters and all.

Sitting in Pour-Over, drinking coffee, me faking it because I don't drink the stuff, Hernandez cries softly as she recounts the inner tension between being with her family and living her life in the big city. She loved Dallas and the freedom, choices, and opportunities that Presidio could not offer, but she missed the family and community connections. Now, even with the conflicting emotion, there is excitement as she describes the future of Pour-Over-Coffee, of the joy of having people from high school and her neighborhood drop in and welcome her back, and of being with her father (who himself unbidden pops in on our interview, even though the shop is closed) and mother and two younger brothers. But there is still, in her words, a sense of impermanence, a statement that she is taking it one day at a time because she still believes that her life may stretch beyond a town that has no streetlights and no future. The prodigal daughter has returned, but no one knows for sure for how long.

Hernandez is a metaphor for social connection in the US, and indeed for much of the world: the pull of community, family, and meaningful work versus the push of the transitory and technology-driven nature of modern life. The scorecard is unbalanced, but there are strategies to build social and civic connection, to reconnect people when the world is conspiring to pull them apart. Modernity may be winning, but as Hernandez's story shows, not everywhere and not all the time.

———

There is, in fact, a small, probably better described as tiny, social health movement growing in the United States, and elsewhere, a dawning realization that social connection is as critical to health as the food you eat, the exercise you may or may not get, and the health care you receive. There has been attention drawn to the personal and community impact of social connection and loneliness, both from the public health perspective—witness the surgeon general's declaration of a loneliness crisis—and also from the civil society perspective, out of a concern that loneliness and isolation are

fueling our political polarization. This has engendered the appointment of ministers of loneliness in Japan and the UK[2] and encouraged a number of other governments to develop at least embryonic
policies around social health.[3]

I won't say the social health movement in the United States is
moving fast—it's still more of a curiosity than a movement—but
there are interesting, protozoic developments. The founders of Soul-
Cycle have started a gym called Peoplehood where you can work
out your relationship skills by participating in hour-long "gathers"
to share openly and listen deeply, sometimes with strangers and
sometimes with partners. There is also a growing class of connection coaches; one such operation works under names that include
the Platonic Action Lab, the Connection Jet Pack, the Connection
Club, the Unbusy Camp, and the Tab Closing Party (which means, I
think, the tabs on your computer, not the tab at the local bar, which
any social coach would probably recommend keeping open anyway). There is also a nascent social prescribing movement, most
developed in the UK, where it is integrated into the National Health
Service, that encourages doctors and other health professionals to
address loneliness and isolation by connecting patients with community organizations and social engagement activities. There are
plenty of other examples of efforts to support people seeking social
connection, or to help those who don't know they need that support. They are all laudable, but in truth, against a vast canvas of
loneliness and isolation in places like the US, they don't yet count
for much.

What is beginning to fill the space is a new DIY movement
that encourages people to take stock of their own social situation
and act to improve it if they need to. If you read *The Good Life*,

for example, by Mark Schulz and Robert Waldinger—the current deputy director and director of the Harvard Study on Adult Development, respectively—you will get both a primer on their research on the importance of relationships to happiness and health and lots of advice on how to strengthen your relationships with the "person next to you," other family members, and friends.

An even sharper example of the genre is *The Art and Science of Connection* by Kasley Killam, the founder of the Social Health Labs. Killam has taken on the difficult task of helping people evaluate their social health. Physical health has endless metrics, and new tools are popping out every day to help you access relevant data. Social health, on the other hand, is far more slippery, lacking standard evaluative and measurement criteria, or least standard evaluative criteria widely understood by the general public. I qualify it only a bit because there are some research-based questions—how many people you can call in the event of an emergency or whether you have a best friend at work—that can give you insights into the comparative state of your social health,[4] but they are not going to afford anyone a comprehensive picture.

It's a difficult problem. Killam has her own approach to social health called the 5-3-1 rule: Spend time with five people each week, nurture at least three close relationships, and aim for one hour of quality connection time each day. It's a little hokey, but so is ten thousand steps, and at least it starts to get at the challenge of measuring and benchmarking—and creating a framework for action for people who are interested in improving their social health.

Killam offers herself up as a case study in how someone who is not naturally extroverted can build social connections. In her book, she tells the story of her 108-day challenge, which she undertook when she was a student at Queen's University in Canada, and her commitment to embracing a new act of connection every day. She picked 108 because the number holds a special place in Buddhism, literature, mathematics, and astronomy—and also in Chicago Cubs lore. And 108 days is long enough that you might be able to observe changes in your well-being and health.

Sometimes her daily deeds were as modest as striking up a conversation with a neighbor or complimenting a clerk at the grocery store. That may not sound like much, but there is extensive evidence that even fleeting engagements such as talking with a fellow passenger on a commuter train can improve happiness and well-being.[5]

Other days, the connections required more planning and commitment: befriending older women from the nearby retirement home or homeless men from the local shelter, or a deeper and longer conversation with an old friend. And sometimes the daily activities were splashier; on the 100th day, Killam and a friend stood at the entrance of the college library with a sign that announced "Feeling stressed about exams? Have a free hug!" That has all sorts of possibilities for being misinterpreted—my thoughts ping-pong between social media censure and plastic handcuffs—but context matters, and Killam reports being rewarded with hundreds of hugs, as the "energy from so many positive interactions vibrated in every cell of [her] body."

You can create your own 108-day social health marathon, but that's not terribly likely. Most of us are not marathoners when it comes to social health and are unlikely to follow the path that Killam has blazed. Improving social health takes individual attention and commitment, just as any aspect of health does, but we should recognize the challenge when so many of the systems that drive social connection—church, unions, social clubs, in-person work, neighborhoods—are in decline, replaced by solitary activities driven by technology. Just as the advent of fast-food restaurants and ultra-processed foods has created the conditions of our obesity crisis, the rise of personal technologies and the decline in convening organizations have conspired to make it ever more difficult to maintain social health. The only real difference between obesity and loneliness is that there is not even the possibility of a magic pill like Ozempic to bring relief.

Killam boldly predicts that we are at the beginning of a great movement, that social health will become a pillar of personal health in the next five years, drawing as much attention as physical and mental health currently does. I hope that is right. The day may be coming when people track their social health much as they do their steps or share tips on Instagram from the best social coaches. I think it is a possibility, but it is by no means a sure thing. People like Robert Putnam have been sounding the alarm about waning social capital and social connection for a quarter century, and we have still been going the wrong way. In the battle between human connection and technology, the score is Steve Jobs one, Robert Putnam zero—and that's being kind to Putnam.

Perhaps, though, when people understand the relationship of social connection to their own healthy longevity, then things will change. There is precedent. Exercise was not so long ago largely the province of weirdos, so much so that in 1968, Senator Strom Thurmond, then one of the most prominent public officials in the country, was stopped by police in Greenville, South Carolina, for the suspicious activity of jogging.[6] Today, there are times when I can look out my front window and see more runners, bikers, and power walkers than cars. Massive industries have grown up around exercise, and social norms have evolved in favor of fitness, so perhaps that can happen with social health as well.

But even fitness is a cautionary tale. We may be more fitness-conscious than in years past, but we are not more fit. Scientists have estimated that Americans' resting metabolic rate—the amount of calories that are burned when the body is at rest—has fallen roughly six percent since 1820, which translates to the equivalent of almost thirty minutes of exercise per day.[7] The decline in the resting metabolic rate is a direct reflection of decreased physical activity over time. You might be startled by this since the Americans of that era had not yet experienced the joys of Tae Bo or the wisdom of Kayla Itsines, but neither had they discovered cars, DoorDash, Zoom, and so many other technologies that have reduced walking, movement, and physical labor.

———

Convincing people that they should tend to their social health is a critical step in supporting healthy longevity. It is, after all, one of the principal goals of this book. But it's not enough. There will be the outliers, the Kasley Killams who will hand out fifty helium balloons to passersby in downtown Toronto, just as there are people who stick to the most rigorous diets. But that's not most people. The rest of us need a cultural context that supports social connection along with opportunities for connection that are easy to access and naturally occurring. Just as we need an adequate supply of healthy foods or a network of gyms, we need a new social infrastructure.

Without it, some people will still flourish, but the majority of people will be at risk of being left behind, the next victims of the loneliness epidemic. Having an effective social framework means having easily accessible opportunities for connection, enabling us to find purpose and stay engaged as we age. The societies that I have profiled in this book have succeeded in part because they have invested in creating a social infrastructure for older (and younger) adults, so that there are multiple ways to stay connected, active, and purposeful. Learning opportunities in Korea, work in Japan, or volunteer service in Italy are all examples of governments and communities coming together to create social infrastructure that supports healthy aging.

The concept of social infrastructure may be an unfamiliar one, but think of it as you might think of food infrastructure. Most everyone understands the basic nutritional maxim of "you are what you eat" and that there are choices to be made between foods that are good for your health and others that are less healthy but may have advantages in terms of cost, taste, or convenience. It's a choice that we make every day, every meal, but if you live in a food swamp (a place saturated with fast food and ultra-processed food options) or a food desert (an area that lacks any healthy food choices), then the choices are more theoretical than real. It is still possible to overcome those grocery limitations and make healthy eating decisions, but realistically most people won't, as the epidemic of obesity, diabetes, and heart disease in some communities can attest. That's the consequence of a food infrastructure that delivers choice to some people and not to others.

We are increasingly living in social deserts. Of course you can overcome that limitation, but we are ultimately products of our social environment and the social cues that society gives us. The good news is that the converse is true: When you create a strong social infrastructure, good health can follow. I saw that in Co-op City in the Bronx, though I didn't have the vocabulary to describe it that way at the time.

If you've ever driven on the Cross Bronx Expressway on the way to New England, you've passed Co-op City, a mini city all its own consisting of thirty-five high-rise buildings with more than fifteen thousand units, as well as a small number of townhouse blocks. Built in the 1960s on the site of a failed amusement park called Freedomland USA, Co-op City was the largest and most ambitious effort to create affordable workforce housing in New York City.[8] Co-op City owns many "largest" medals. It is the largest cooperative housing project in the United States and the largest NORC—naturally occurring retirement community—in the world. And like Presidio County, life expectancy in Co-op City is much higher than geography suggests it should be.

Income, health care, nutrition, and exercise in Co-op City differ little from the shorter-lived neighborhoods surrounding it. What is different are the levels of social connection and neighborhood support, which are extensive in Co-op City. It's not that people in Co-op City are naturally friendly or socially adventurous, but they live in a community that supports connection. Unlike most of New York City, apartments in Co-op City are both generous in size and affordable, less than a third of the average rent in Manhattan. Because of this, people who are lucky enough to get an apartment—there is a long waiting list—tend to settle in and never move. People age in place and aspire to pass on their apartments to their children—sometimes legally, sometimes not. The stability of the population means that even in famously unfriendly New York there is neighborhood and community: People know one another, they form lasting friendships and relationships, they look after one another, and they support one another as they age—and over time they build community organizations that deepen ties even further. Old-timers—and there are plenty of them—will tell you that it's not like the old days, and to a certain extent that may be right. The original settlers had a natural bonding experience from creating the place—and from winning the rent strikes of the 1970s—and more recent transplants simply haven't had as much time to gel in the same way, but they will have that chance over the coming decades to forge their own brand of community. In Co-op City, social connection is a product of a stable housing infrastructure, and there is a big health dividend that comes from that.

If you wanted to find two places on the map of the US that are diametrically opposite, you could do worse than stabbing at Presidio and Co-op City: one a quiet, rural outpost across a bridge from Mexico, the other a high-rise haven in the loudest, most congested, and most frenetic city in the country. But both are public health case studies because they have highly developed social health infrastructures—conditions that make it easier, and to a certain extent unavoidable, for people to stay connected, engaged, and part of a larger community. In Presidio, the social infrastructure is a product of social norms and familial customs. In Co-op City, it is a result of public policy—development of the project was underwritten in part by New York State tax incentives—and a social commitment to quality affordable housing, a commitment that has unfortunately been eroded by time, politics, and economics. If we are to have more Presidios and more Co-op Cities in the US and elsewhere, we will have to be far more intentional as a society in creating the preconditions for social connection and community.

I thought a lot about Co-op City when I visited the Queenstown Health District in Singapore. The Queenstown neighborhood bears a passing physical resemblance to Co-op City, from the warren of high-rise buildings to the green spaces that snake through them. And the similarity does not end there, as both places have built the foundation for healthier, longer life. To be fair, the term "social infrastructure" would likely have been puzzling to the founders of Co-op City, but they almost certainly had an innate sense of the value of community, if not the direct link it has to healthy longevity. Queenstown, on the other hand, is intentional about social infrastructure, even if John Wong and his fellow architects don't use that exact phrase. More than any other place that I have been to or researched, the Queenstown effort leverages a vast array of tools—intergenerational housing, learning programs, social clubs, work, family ties—to create a web of connections to help people of all ages, but especially older adults, stay active, engaged, and able to live lives full of meaning. You can be lonely in Queenstown, as you can be anywhere, but the idea is to make it as hard as possible by living in a place where people are constantly interacting, looking after one another, and encouraging everyone to participate in a long list of activities. That's social infrastructure.

Unfortunately, the social infrastructure in many places, including the United States, is decaying, the product of long neglect and disinterest. Declines in club participation, political activism, and personal friendships and increases in social media obsession are all examples of a society defined by loneliness and isolation. And institutions such as churches and unions that have historically created the contours of our communities and fostered social connections are all in long-term decline and not likely to rebound anytime soon.[9]

The social infrastructure of the future will look different from that of the past, and institutions from cities to universities to businesses will have to play a role in fostering social health. There are some green sprouts: Look at the rise in multigenerational households and changes in social norms around co-living, for instance, and clear opportunities around older workers and older volunteers. As the surgeon general's report highlighted, there is growing awareness of the risks of loneliness to personal and collective health, but progress requires new efforts and new investments.

If you've gotten this far in the book, you probably care about the issue, so perhaps more persuasion on this topic is not necessary. But if it is, we should understand that there is a cost well beyond health. A socially isolated and lonely society is an angry society, and we are seeing the cost of that in ways too numerous and frankly too depressing to fully enumerate here. It's reflected in higher rates of suicide, depression, and drug abuse, as well as higher rates of political polarization. And it is not just the fact that people disagree with one another—that's a feature of democratic society—but the heightened mistrust and fear that comes when civic life is not mediated by real human relationships across political divides.

—

In much of this book, I've toggled back and forth on the story of personal health (what you can do for yourself and your family) and public health (how to address the broader concerns and implications of an aging population). Those concepts are linked—public health is the sum of our collective personal well-being—but it is also true that the policies and approaches between the two are rather different. In the concluding part of each chapter, I've focused on personal health. But here to complete the book, I'm going to focus more on the public side of the story, the things we need to do to build a social health infrastructure to support communal health.

When Singapore began to get serious about healthy aging, it launched Age Well SG—a coordinated program of the Ministry of Health, the Ministry of National Development, and the Ministry of Transportation—to build a social health infrastructure to keep older adults active, engaged, and purposeful, and it backed it up with hundreds of millions of dollars in investment. And it has continued to fund that commitment to this day. When I talk with people about Singapore and healthy aging, they sometimes dismiss the country as an example because it is wealthy and can afford to make investments. But Singapore has made those investments not because it can afford them. It has made those investments because it can't afford not to make them. The health care costs of a sickly aging population are simply staggering. In the United States, people over the age of sixty-five account for roughly $1.7 trillion annually in health care spending (about 6 percent of our entire GDP right there), roughly double the per capita basis of the population as a whole. The driver of this is not just older people as a group, but a subset of the older population that is in poor or fair health. More than $800 billion is spent on just 10 percent of the sixty-five and older population.[10] Of course we will spend a disproportionate amount of health care dollars on an aging population, but if we were to keep more older adults active and engaged, we would save hundreds of billions of dollars every year.

And it's not just the economics of it all. Successful aging is a reflection of a healthy society, one that supports the development of its citizens from the earliest years to the last ones. You simply can't have a society that ages well if people in the second half of life are not supported, not engaged with their families, friends, colleagues, and communities, and not afforded opportunities to work, learn, and contribute. We are far from living in that society, but there is a path forward, and below I present seven keys to building a new social infrastructure. In developing them, I've been inspired by the work of the Stanford Center on Longevity (SCL), one of the world's leading centers of learning and research on longevity and aging. More than any other place that I know of, SCL has worked to shift the conversation from the problem of "what do we do with all these old people?" to the question of how we can create a society where longer life is healthier and more productive, and where the gift of longer life is available to more people. But even more than SCL, I've been inspired by seeing these social investments work in communities around the world, giving more people the opportunity for longer, healthier lives than ever before. Some of these ideas are programmatic, some are cultural, and some are a mix, but together they can help us build social health and healthier, longer lives.

Build intergenerational relationships the Singaporean way. Evolutionary biology is an amazing thing. For almost all of history, intergenerational relationships have been a natural and necessary part of human existence. Generations stayed together so that older people could protect and nurture younger generations, a role critical to the future of the species. Even today, living near grandmothers confers evolutionary benefits in terms of more and healthier children.[11]

For a century, we have been fighting evolutionary biology, and biology is punishing us with an epidemic of loneliness and poor health. Maybe we will be recoded differently in the future, if we have a few million years to spare. But for the moment we are better off acknowledging the critical role that intergenerational relationships play in human flourishing and lean into it as a foundational element of social health infrastructure.

No country has done more to support intergenerational relationships than Singapore, because it views them as central to supporting healthy living. The strategy is integrated into housing and tax policy, how social and volunteer organizations work, in business policies, and in public health communications. Not all aspects of the Singapore approach will fit more individualistic societies—Americans are not likely to substantially restrict housing options for single people under thirty-five—but we can certainly try to emulate its norm-setting in favor of intergenerational support and nationally appropriate policies and investments to bring the generations back together.

Support a physical infrastructure that connects people as in Spain. Buffalo, New York, is known mostly for urban decay, snowfall accumulation, and football futility. But once upon a time, it was considered one of the loveliest cities in the world. Designed by Frederick Law Olmsted, the renowned landscape architect and creator of Central Park in New York City, Buffalo was called the "Emerald Necklace," a reference to the ribbons of parks and greenery that crowned the city. Central to the design was the Humboldt Parkway, a two-mile-long, tree-lined boulevard that linked the two largest city parks. Generations of families walked, biked, played, and connected in the broad shade of the parkway.

In 1957, Buffalo plowed under the Humboldt Parkway in favor of the Kensington Expressway, a trenched highway that would ferry people at high speeds between downtown and the new suburbs rising to the east. In favoring suburbia and high-speed transportation, Buffalo condemned a string of urban neighborhoods to decades of social isolation and poor health because residents no longer had any places to safely gather. The boarded homes, soot-encrusted storefronts, and nosediving health stats are a testament to what happens when community is lost.

Barcelona has taken a different approach with the creation of the superblocks, which close areas to vehicular traffic and create more public space for people to gather and build social health. It is a design that declares cities are for people, not cars, and it is a specific recognition of the importance of design to healthy living. In return, Barcelona has been rewarded with an improvement in measures of livability, environmental quality, and health.[12] It is not a simple thing to do, and even earlier, grander plans for Barcelona have been scuttled by political reality, but the rewards in terms of personal and community health can be immense. Each community will have its own approach. Los Angeles will be different from Barcelona, but we will go further if we acknowledge the link between the built environment and social health.

Support positive views of aging as in Japan. There is a lot to dislike about ageism, but all the problems with it are magnified by the fact that ageism remains socially acceptable, a fact you can confirm for yourself by perusing social media for the routine dismissal of the views of people just because they are perceived as too old. It's an underappreciated environmental cost, and it leaves older people thinking that they are less worthy, less valuable, and a burden on society.

In 2021, the World Health Organization launched a global campaign to combat ageism. It was in a difficult context, coming on the heels of a pandemic that pitted generations against each other, but the message was nonetheless relevant: *Age should not define us.* A seventy-five-year-old man might be in very good physical shape, or he might be in rapid physical decline. His mental acuity might be enhanced by a lifetime of learning, or he might be in the throes of dementia. Heterogeneity is possible at any life stage, but it compounds as we age, which means age as a developmental marker loses potency over the course of a lifetime. Knowing that someone is fifteen will tell you a lot about their stage of physical and cognitive development. Knowing someone is seventy will tell you far less.

We should all take a page from societies like Japan that have strongly developed respect for older people and are creating opportunities for them to find value, purpose, and meaning in later life. But we should go beyond Japan and recognize that ageism is not just a one-way street. Younger people are also swept up in ageist tropes. Rejecting all forms of ageism in favor of cooperation among the generations will only increase the opportunity for social health and connection.

Learn throughout life like in Korea. Structurally, our education system has changed little in the last century. Many colleges and universities make the timeliness of their approach a point of pride; a professor at Columbia Business School once smugly told me that elite universities would never change, because students would still clamor to attend them simply because of the reputational halo. The unbending nature of our educational system and our elite institutions is disheartening at a time of rapid social change and when people increasingly need access to lifelong learning to stay economically competitive and healthy.

Educational attainment has come to divide our society, distinguishing those who can anticipate long, healthy lives from those who cannot. Americans with a four-year college degree live about nine years longer than those without a high school diploma, roughly the same gap overall that exists between the United States and Turkmenistan. Postsecondary education equates to more job opportunities, more economic security, and better health, and it increasingly is a bigger cleavage in American life than race, geography, or gender.

Total spending for public elementary and secondary education in the US is roughly $768 billion.[13] Spending by colleges and universities is in the same ballpark, a little over $700 billion. In contrast, the federal government contributes about $675 million to states for adult education.[14] There is nuance to those numbers, but nuance doesn't matter too much when spending for education before age twenty-one is roughly two thousand times what it is for all the years that follow. Creating a true lifelong learning environment requires a much larger investment by society in making adult learning widely available and affordable.

Change may come slowly in academia but not in Korea. There are now approximately 170 lifelong learning cities in Korea, encompassing well over three-quarters of the population, and Korean universities have begun to rethink how to serve learners over the entire life course, not just in the small number of years between high school and work. The reinvention of learning into a lifetime endeavor is one of the most significant changes in education this century and should be a model for the rest of the world.

Work more years, with greater flexibility, as in Japan. The success of Japan in increasing the participation of older workers in the labor force has been due not to the blunt edge of retirement rules but the fine point of creating a new work culture—one in which older workers aspire to keep working and companies scramble to accommodate them. It is often assumed that changing retirement rules and payouts will naturally result in changing work practices, but recent history has shown us that when workers want out—or when employers want them out—retirement rules be damned. The US, for instance, has changed Social Security payout rules numerous times over the last thirty years in order to incentivize working longer, but the actual retirement age hasn't shifted much in sixty years. It must drive economists crazy.

Japan is forging a new compact with older workers to make later-life work more attractive, more flexible, and more closely connected to health. There are many elements to this compact, from increased training to more flexible work rules to providing a glide path for people nearing retirement who do not want to simply fall off a work cliff. Flexible working hours are among the most attractive measures to create a new phase of work that combines elements of retirement and productivity. The idea is highly coveted by American workers. About 40 percent of older Americans say they would be willing to take a 10 percent reduction in hourly wage, and about 20 percent would be willing to take a 20 percent reduction in hourly wage to work part-time, or work under a flexible schedule.[15] None of that happens without employers understanding the current and future role of older workers in the labor force and without workers understanding the nexus between continuing work and good health. Japan has understood this well before the rest of us.

Favor in-person activities as in Italy. Our ancestors sought connection through physical proximity because there was safety in numbers. Being alone signals danger, and no amount of Zooming or TikToks will relieve the heightened stress of social isolation. Unfortunately, we live in an age of blossoming aloneness, and it's getting worse. Today, Gen Z gets one thousand fewer hours of in-person connection every year compared to previous generations.[16] That translates to three fewer hours every day. It's a scary situation in an era when technology is increasingly keeping us apart instead of bringing us together as technologists once promised.

Social health requires physical proximity, and Italy has made that a priority in the post-COVID-19 era. It's influenced, no doubt, by a culture that has long celebrated physical togetherness at family dinners, at group events, or in the physical intimacy of relationships. Increasingly, Italians, and their cultural cousins in Spain, are further supporting togetherness by underwriting cultural events, expanding volunteer opportunities,[17] and enlarging community centers that naturally bring people and generations together. It's an old model, but one that is increasingly critical in a digitally absorbed world.

Redefine the retirement years as an encore career, like people in Singapore, Japan, Korea, Spain, and Italy all do. And this brings us full circle, back to Sarah and Jay and Table 23: the promise of a bright future versus the beginning of the end. The people making big plans and the people shelving old ones. It's a matter of perspective. Everyone at Table 23 has a good shot at another twenty years of good health. Not everyone will get there, or at least that's what the actuarial tables tell us, but the odds are significantly enhanced by embracing the opportunity of these extra years.

If you frame it right, most older adults will see the possibilities. In 2003, two researchers, Helene Fung of the Chinese University of Hong Kong and Laura Carstensen of Stanford, showed two groups of participants—one younger and one older—two advertisements for a new camera. Both ads featured an identical set of photos of nature, travel, and relaxation, but one was captioned "capture those special moments," and the other was captioned "capture the unexplored world." The older group favored the slogan about special moments, while the younger group gravitated toward the unexplored world. But when the older group was primed with the idea that they could live another twenty years longer in good health, they reversed course and chose the unexplored world, drawn to the idea that the future was not about remembering but creating.[18]

It's a different script for the years past sixty than the one we are used to. It is not hyperbole to say that our collective future hinges upon our ability to reimagine ourselves as contributors, not takers— as part of the future, not a legacy of the past. That is the promise of greater longevity and the path to a healthier, longer life.

All the countries I have profiled here invest in helping older adults envision a new future—and plan for it. Whether that is the Silver Jinzai organization in Japan, lifelong learning cities in Korea, or volunteer centers in Italy, there are myriad resources to help older adults imagine and plan the next twenty years, or even the next thirty. It can be work, but it doesn't have to be. It can be volunteering, intergenerational care, or lifelong learning, or some combination of all of the above: The path to purpose and connection is wide. But all of these approaches are linked by the belief that older people are not just marking time toward an inevitable end. They are part of a generation that has important things to offer society. No one has to say it, but there is an unspoken assumption that the years in front can be—really need to be—as productive and useful as the ones that are in our immediate rearview. This is the promise of healthy to 100, and it is a possibility that is open to everyone at Table 23—and the rest of us too—if we can imagine that future.

ACKNOWLEDGMENTS

A LL BOOKS ARE solitary and communal experiences wrapped together, but a book like this especially requires a huge amount of active support: from friends, colleagues, experts, and even complete strangers. I wish I could thank everyone who helped me along the way—I wish I had kept an accurate list—but here's a start:

In my mind, this book became real the day I stood in our kitchen and disclosed to Beth my plans to trundle off to Asia and Europe for three months, leaving her with a twelve-hour-a-day job and a twenty-four-hour-a-day family to manage by herself. I stood clear of the kitchen knives when I told her, a prudent but fortunately unnecessary precaution, as she has been (mostly) a cheerful and supportive partner in this endeavor.

I'm particularly grateful to Laura Carstensen and the entire team at the Stanford Center on Longevity. Laura has been a teacher and an inspiration to countless people in the field, and like so many of them, I am indebted to her for introducing me to the field of longevity, advising me on this book, and letting me rip off many of her ideas along the way. Anyone who wants to learn more about longevity should check out her writings and the New Map of Life. It's an amazing group at Stanford, and it has been a privilege to work with David Pagano, Laura Tejada, Nikki Tran Duff, Jackie Macdonald, Joleen Castro, Yochai Shavit, and Marie Conley-Smith. And I am saving the best for last, as I will always be thankful for the friendship and support of Martha Deevy, who has been my partner (and occasional taskmaster) in longevity since I started working in the field some eight years ago.

My colleagues on the *Century Lives* podcast and at the Longevity Project have been an enormous source of ideas and support. Kerry Thompson, Kate Rarey, and Erin Bump in particular, with special thanks to Kerry for helping to plan out the overseas investigations for this book.

There are many in the field of longevity and aging who have given me incredible feedback for the book. Starting with Marc Freedman, who has been a great friend and advisor and who provided important feedback here, especially on the intergenerational topic. I am also deeply grateful to Bradley Schurman, the author of *The Super Age*. I had never met Bradley, never even emailed with him, before I reached out to pick his brain for the book, and yet he jumped right into brainstorming with me on the book, advising on where to go and who to talk to, and making introductions across the world. Some of the best stories in this book are here only because Bradley helped me find them. There have been many other people in the field who have influenced me—either through their writings, their speeches, or even just in conversation—including Paul Irving, Andrew Scott, and Chip Conley, just to name a few.

Reporting overseas is hard, language barriers are harder. I was fortunate to work with great translators and fixers everywhere I went (thank you, Anthony Kuhn of NPR, for helping me find great people). In Japan, Takehiro Masutomo was super, as were Jinseo Park in

Korea and Lourdes Pérez Munilla in Spain. In Singapore, John Wong from the National University of Singapore, whom you met in the book, was extraordinarily helpful in not just spending time with me but also suggesting and arranging other meetings and interviews. Lydia Cheung and Ng Zi En, who for some reason dubbed themselves as my "Mini-Friends," served as my minders in Singapore and were a delight. I did largely manage to navigate Italy on my own but wouldn't have been able to do so without the insights and assistance of Paolo Compostella and Matteo Martone of APCO.

The list of people I interviewed for this book is too long to reasonably set forth here, but I am grateful to all who gave up their time to talk with me. It is worth calling out a number of people who went above and beyond, not just in making themselves available but offering ideas and facilitating other meetings as well. In Korea, Ayleen Jung at the Seoul 50 Plus Foundation and Kyung Hi Kim at Kyungnam University were incredibly helpful. In Spain, I am grateful to Juan Martín from CENIE, who welcomed me to the Spain-Japan Summit on Longevity, Elisa Sala in Barcelona, and especially to Pablo García Vivanco in Ourense, who hosted me for a memorable (and exhausting) day of interviews, meetings, meals, and a dip in the thermal baths that are a delight of the region. In Italy, a special thanks to Marisa Gaiardelli from Pro Senectute in Omegna. In Singapore it seems like everyone is a longevity enthusiast, and I could have interviewed the whole city, but special thanks to Mary Ann Tsao of the Tsao Foundation, who squeezed me in for a great conversation between hosting a student reception for Wellesley College and an unrelated dinner party, and the team at St. John's-St. Margaret's who made time for me on a Friday and then even more time on Saturday morning after I insisted on coming back to learn more.

Thanks to my editors at PublicAffairs, Emily Taber and Colleen Lawrie, for partnering with me on the book, and especially to Emily, who took over when Colleen went out on maternity leave and demonstrated an unfortunate skill in calling me out when my treasured stories became too long and unwieldy. I am still reeling from losing the story of me and Nate at the Fountain of Youth Archeological Park in St. Augustine, Florida. I still love the story and am happy to tell it to anyone who wants to drop by.

And special thanks to my agent, Gillian MacKenzie, who for reasons that remain a mystery to me has continued to believe in me as a writer and serve as an impassioned advocate on my behalf.

Ultimately, this book is about relationships and friendships that sustain you through life—and for me, through the book writing process as well. There are so many people in my life: friends, family, colleagues, who have played a silent but critical role in the development of this book. They didn't have anything to do specifically with the book (though a shout-out to my sister-in-law, Liz Stern, who was the source of the best chapter heading in the book), but they have had everything to do with making life meaningful and worthwhile and giving me the impetus and the energy for this book. My fondest wish is that they all live healthy to 100.

NOTES

Introduction

1. "GHE: Life Expectancy and Healthy Life Expectancy," n.d., https://www.who.int /data/gho/data/themes/mortality-and-global-health-estimates/ghe-life-expectancy -and-healthy-life-expectancy#:~:text=Situation%20and%20trends,and%2061.9%20 years%2C%20respectively). The World Health Organization maintains healthy life expectancy data for every country, with highs ranging from roughly seventy-four (Japan) to forty-five (Central African Republic).

2. Katharina Buchholz, "Where People Are Working Beyond 65," *Statista Daily Data*, March 17, 2023, https://www.statista.com/chart/12202/where-people-are-working -beyond-65/#:~:text=There%20is%20a%20huge%20disparity%20in%20labor,force %20%2D%20between%2013%20and%2014%20percent.

3. Robert Waldinger and Marc Schulz, *The Good Life: Lessons from the World's Longest Scientific Study of Happiness* (Simon and Schuster, 2023).

4. "Our Epidemic of Loneliness and Isolation: The U.S. Surgeon General's Advisory on the Healing Effects of Social Connection and Community [Internet]," Office of the Surgeon General, 2023, https://pubmed.ncbi.nlm.nih.gov/37792968/.

5. L. F. Berkman and S. L. Syme, "Social Networks, Host Resistance, and Mortality: A Nine-Year Follow-up Study of Alameda County Residents," *American Journal of Epidemiology* 109, no. 2. (February 1979): 186–204.

6. James S. House, Karl R. Landis, and Debra Umberson, "Social Relationships and Health," *Science* 241, no. 4865 (July 29, 1988): 540–545, https://doi.org/10.1126 /science.3399889.

7. Waldinger and Schulz, *The Good Life: Lessons from the World's Longest Scientific Study of Happiness*, 46.

8. "Our Epidemic of Loneliness and Isolation: The U.S. Surgeon General's Advisory on the Healing Effects of Social Connection and Community," 24.

9. Álvaro Sánchez, "The Spaniards Who Are Breaking the 100-Year Age Barrier," *EL PAÍS English*, February 16, 2016, https://english.elpais.com/elpais/2016/02/08 /inenglish/1454924775_816830.html.

10. John T. Cacioppo, Stephanie Cacioppo, John P. Capitanio, and Steven W. Cole. "The Neuroendocrinology of Social Isolation." *Annual Review of Psychology* 66 (August 23, 2014): 733–767, https://doi.org/10.1146/annurev-psych-010814-015240.

11. "Our Epidemic of Loneliness and Isolation: The U.S. Surgeon General's Advisory on the Healing Effects of Social Connection and Community," 24–34.

12. Raj Chetty et al., "The Association Between Income and Life Expectancy in the United States," *JAMA* 315, no. 16 (April 26, 2016): 1750–1766.

13. Given the movement of population back and forth between Presidio County in Texas and the neighboring state of Chihuahua in Mexico, it is possible that some of the remarkable life expectancy numbers are due in part to inconsistent recordkeeping between the two jurisdictions. Just as the data behind the Blue Zones have been put into question, so should we cast a skeptical eye toward any data that breaks with familiar evidentiary patterns. I remain both impressed with health in Presidio but also open to the possibility that the data does not show the full picture. Whatever the peculiarities of the data in Presidio, the town and county are still an important reflection of the Hispanic Paradox, which is well-documented across a much broader set of communities in the United States.

14. "GHE: Life Expectancy and Healthy Life Expectancy," n.d.

15. Robert D. Putnam, *Bowling Alone: The Collapse and Revival of American Community* (Simon and Schuster, 2000).

16. Quoted in Jeevan Vasagar, *Lion City: Singapore and the Invention of Modern Asia* (Little, Brown UK, 2021). *Lion City* provides a fascinating general account from the local *Financial Times* correspondent of Singapore's rapid economic and social ascendency over the last half century.

17. Stanford Center on Longevity, "The New Map of Life," April 2022, https://longevity.stanford.edu/the-new-map-of-life-initiative/.

18. United Nations, "Global Issues: Ageing," n.d., https://www.un.org/en/global-issues/ageing#:~:text=The%20world's%20population%20is%20ageing,for%20a%20growing%20older%20population.

19. Kaare Christensen et al., "Ageing Populations: The Challenges Ahead," *The Lancet* 374, no. 9696: 1196–1208. But also see Jay Olshansky et al., "Ageing and Health," *The Lancet* 375, no. 9708: 25, for a more recent analysis that life expectancy growth may be approaching a natural limit.

20. Central Intelligence Agency, "Country Comparisons—Total Fertility Rate," n.d., https://www.cia.gov/the-world-factbook/field/total-fertility-rate/country-comparison/.

21. There is just not much out there on Diamond Lil McConnell, I am sad to say. She deserves more. The thin history that does exist suggests that she was a practicing doctor in Chicago who decided to seek her fortune in the Yukon. Tales of her time in the Yukon, most likely exaggerated, are recorded in her book *The Tragedy of the Klondike: This Book of Travels Gives the True Facts of What Took Place in the Goldfields Under British Rule*. From the Yukon, her travels are uncertain, some sources placing her in California, others in Zimbabwe (in an area then called Southern Rhodesia). But we do know from newspapers of the time that she arrived in St. Augustine in August 1904 with tales of husbands left behind and a diamond in a front tooth.

22. Bradley Schurman, *The Super Age: Decoding Our Demographic Destiny* (Harper Business, 2022), 41.

23. Venki Ramakrishnan, *Why We Die: The New Science of Aging and the Quest for Immortality* (William Morrow, 2024), 3. Mark Oliver, "The First Emperor of China Took an 'Elixir of Immortality' Made of Mercury and It Killed Him," Ancient Origins, September 3, 2022, https://www.ancient-origins.net/weird-facts/elixir-life-0017223.

24. Schurman, *The Super Age*, 42.

25. Saul Justin Newman, "Supercentenarian and Remarkable Age Records Exhibit Patterns Indicative of Clerical Errors and Pension Fraud," *bioRxiv (Cold Spring Harbor Laboratory)*, July 16, 2019, https://doi.org/10.1101/704080.

Chapter 1: *Hurry, Hurry*

1. "Kyungnam University Website," Kyungnam University, https://www.kyungnam.ac.kr/sites/en/index..do. Kyungnam University has a student body of about ten thousand students, spread over six colleges.

2. "Credential Confusion: New Report Identifies More Than One Million Credentials Offered in the U.S. Across a Maze of Nearly 60,000 Providers," Credential Engine, December 7, 2022, https://credentialengine.org/2022/12/07/credential-confusion-new -report-identifies-more-than-one-million-credentials-offered-in-the-u-s-across-a -maze-of-nearly-60000-providers/#:~:text=Credential%20Confusion:%20New%20 Report%20Identifies,traditional%20institutions%20of%20higher%20education.

3. John Bynner, "Whatever Happened to Lifelong Learning? And Does It Matter?," *Journal of the British Academy* 5 (March 21, 2017): 61–89, https://doi.org/10.5871/jba /005.061.

4. "Strengthening the Governance of Skill Systems," OECD, March 27, 2020, https://www.oecd.org/en/publications/strengthening-the-governance-of-skills-systems _3a4bb6ea-en.html.

5. Sam Kim/Bloomberg, "Seoul to Offer Cash for Vasectomy Reversals in Bid to Boost Languishing Birth Rate," *TIME*, May 28, 2024, https://time.com/6982555/south -korea-seoul-subsidizes-reverse-vasectomy-tubectomy-low-birth-rate/. The Seoul city budget also includes funding for underwriting hospitalization costs for pregnant women over the age of thirty-five and subsidies for wedding venues. None of it has worked in a material way yet, though birth rates in Korea did rebound modestly in 2023, the first recorded increase in a decade.

6. Jung Min-Ho, "Sales of Pet Strollers Surpass Baby Strollers for 1st Time," *The Korea Times*, December 27, 2023, https://www.koreatimes.co.kr/www/culture /2024/09/135_365753.html.

7. "Strengthening the Governance of Skill Systems," OECD, March 27, 2020.

8. Brittne Kakulla, "Lifelong Learning Among 45+ Adults," AARP, March 25, 2022, https://doi.org/10.26419/res.00526.001.

9. "What Is Cognitive Reserve?," Harvard Health, February 1, 2024, https://www .health.harvard.edu/mind-and-mood/what-is-cognitive-reserve.

10. David A. Snowdon, "Healthy Aging and Dementia: Findings from the Nun Study," *Annals of Internal Medicine* 139, no. 5_Part_2 (September 2, 2003): 450, https:// doi.org/10.7326/0003-4819-139-5_part_2-200309021-00014.

11. Michael D. Lemonick and Alice Park Mankato, "The Nun Study: How One Scientist and 678 Sisters Are Helping Unlock the Secrets of Alzheimer's," *TIME*, May 14, 2001, https://time.com/archive/6953351/the-nun-study-how-one-scientist-and-678 -sisters-are-helping-unlock-the-secrets-of-alzheimers/.

12. Richard G. Rogers et al., "Educational Degrees and Adult Mortality Risk in the United States," *Biodemography and Social Biology* 56, no. 1 (April 23, 2010): 80–99, https://doi.org/10.1080/19485561003727372.

13.   Panos Photopoulos et al., "Remote and In-Person Learning: Utility Versus Social Experience," *SN Computer Science* 4, no. 2 (December 21, 2022), https://doi .org/10.1007/s42979-022-01539-6.

14. Sebastiano Benasso et al., *Landscapes of Lifelong Learning Policies Across Europe: Comparative Case Studies* (Palgrave Macmillan, 2022).

15. "Case Study: Lifelong Learning in Korea," in OECD Skills Studies, March 27, 2020, https://doi.org/10.1787/cd2b486a-en.

16. "Background: 50+ in Seoul, Korea," Seoul 50 Plus Foundation, n.d., https://50plus.or.kr/org/eng.do. Despite the "Foundation" in its name, the organization is a government agency, part of the Seoul city government. Because of that, the 50 Plus Foundation has seen its mission evolve as political control has moved from one administration to the next. While the focus has always remained on the challenges of midlife, the foundation's original focus on the whole person—purpose, social connection, and planning for the second half of life—has narrowed to building skills and reemployment opportunities. Some of the original functions have gradually transferred to its sister organization, the Seoul Lifelong Learning Institute.

17. "Lifelong Learning and Technology," Pew Research Center, March 22, 2016, https://www.pewresearch.org/internet/2016/03/22/lifelong-learning-and-technology/.

18. Kakulla, "Lifelong Learning Among 45+ Adults," March 25, 2022.

19. "History of U3A Worldwide," U3A Sunshine Coast, n.d., https://u3asunshine .org.au/newweb/history-of-u3a-worldwide/. "U3a—About Us," University of the Third Age, n.d., https://www.u3a.org.uk/about.

20. "Osher Lifelong Learning Institutes," The Bernard Osher Foundation, 2005, https://www.osherfoundation.org/olli.html.

21. Viji Diane Kannan and Peter J. Veazie, "US Trends in Social Isolation, Social Engagement, and Companionship—Nationally and by Age, Sex, Race/Ethnicity, Family Income, and Work Hours, 2003–2020," *SSM—Population Health* 21 (March 2023): 101331, https://doi.org/10.1016/j.ssmph.2022.101331.

22. "Kwŏn Kŭn," Wikipedia, October 26, 2024, https://en.wikipedia.org/wiki/Kw %C5%8Fn_K%C5%ADn. Gwon Geun, also translated as Kwon Kun, was a fourteenth-century Neo-Confucian scholar at the beginning of the Josean era, a dynastic kingdom that ruled Korea for five hundred years.

23. In Tak Kwon et al., "Becoming a Lifelong Learning City: Lessons from a Provincial City in South Korea," journal article, n.d., https://files.eric.ed.gov/fulltext /ED570514.pdf.

24. Chris Impey, "Massive Online Open Courses See Exponential Growth During COVID-19 Pandemic," The Conversation, July 23, 2020, https://theconversation.com/massive-online-open-courses-see-exponential-growth-during-covid-19-pandemic-141859.

25. Momna Azmat and Ayesha Ahmad, "Lack of Social Interaction in Online Classes During COVID-19," *Journal of Materials and Environmental Science* 13, no. 2 (March 5, 2022): 185–196, https://www.jmaterenvironsci.com/Document/vol13/vol13_N2/JMES-2022-13015-Azmat.pdf.

26. Nicole Goodkind, "Some Colleges Cost $95,000 per Year, and They're Only Getting More Expensive. Here's Why," CNN Business, July 16, 2023, https://www.cnn.com/2023/07/16/investing/curious-consumer-college-cost/index.html.

Chapter 2: *Bismarck's Revenge*

1. Deutsche Welle, "Explained: How Japan Keeps Its Elderly Employed and Active," Frontline, October 16, 2021, https://frontline.thehindu.com/dispatches/explained-how-japan-keeps-its-elderly-employed-and-active/article37017427.ece.

2. Hitoshi Nakano (chairman of Silver Jinzai in Fukuoka, Japan) in discussion with the author, March 18, 2024.

3. Yohei Matsuo, "Japan Retirement Trends: Job-Seeking Seniors Double in 10 Years," *Nikkei Asia*, January 4, 2024, https://asia.nikkei.com/Spotlight/Work/Japan-retirement-trends-job-seeking-seniors-double-in-10-years.

4. "A Third of Japanese People Aged 70 to 74 Still in the Workforce," nippon.com, October 10, 2023, https://www.nippon.com/en/japan-data/h01797/.

5. "2024 Workforce State of Mind," Headspace, n.d., https://get.headspace.com/2024-workforce-state-of-mind#WSOM-form.

6. Pamela Druckerman, "Why the French Want to Stop Working," *The Atlantic*, January 25, 2023, https://www.theatlantic.com/ideas/archive/2023/01/paris-france-retirement-pension-reform-protests/672824/.

7. Sarah Laskow, "How Retirement Was Invented," *The Atlantic*, October 24, 2014, https://www.theatlantic.com/business/archive/2014/10/how-retirement-was-invented/381802/.

8. Angela M. Antonelli, "The Aging of America: A Changing Picture of Work and Retirement," Georgetown Center for Retirement Initiatives, March 2018, https://cri.georgetown.edu/the-aging-of-america-a-changing-picture-of-work-and-retirement/. The average age of retirement has bounced around for years, from peaks around sixty-eight in the 1950s to lows around fifty-seven in the 1990s. Since the 1990s, the effective age of retirement has gradually risen to its current level of sixty-two, still well below mid-century levels.

9. Schurman, *The Super Age*.

10. Héctor García and Francesc Miralles, *Ikigai: The Japanese Secret to a Long and Happy Life* (Penguin, 2017).

11. Philippe Debroux, "Employment of Senior Workers in Japan," *Contemporary Japan* 34, no. 1 (March 15, 2022): 58–86, https://doi.org/10.1080/18692729.2022.2028

228. Yu Korekawa, "Employment of Older Persons in Japan: Perspectives on History, Policy, and the Impact of Technology," Online meeting (Zoom), June 22, 2022.

12. "Percentage of Employees Feeling Severely Insecure and Stressed in their Working Environment in Japan from 1997 to 2022," Statista, January 9, 2024, https://www.statista.com/statistics/623230/japan-stress-at-work/#:~:text=According%20to%20a%20survey%20conducted,in%20their%20current%20working%20situation.

13. Hui Nemeth and Alden Lai, "Japan's Workplace Wellbeing Woes Continue," *Gallup* (blog), September 7, 2023, https://news.gallup.com/opinion/gallup/510257/japan-workplace-wellbeing-woes-continue.aspx.

14. Motokazu Matsui, "Nearly 40% of Japanese Companies Hire People over 70 Years Old," Nikkei Asia, August 13, 2023, https://asia.nikkei.com/Spotlight/Datawatch/Nearly-40-of-Japanese-companies-hire-people-over-70-years-old.

15. Naoko Tochibayashi and Mizuho Ota, "How Companies Are Addressing Workforce Shortages and Employee Satisfaction with Senior Employment in Japan," World Economic Forum, August 15, 2024, https://www.weforum.org/stories/2024/08/how-companies-are-addressing-workforce-shortages-through-senior-employment-in-japan/.

16. Noam Scheiber, "What It Feels Like to Be Washed Up at 35," *The New Republic*, March 23, 2014, https://newrepublic.com/article/117088/silicons-valleys-brutal-ageism.

17. Kumar Mehta, "Older Entrepreneurs Outperform Younger Founders—Shattering Ageism," *Forbes*, August 25, 2022, https://www.forbes.com/sites/kmehta/2022/08/23/older-entrepreneurs-outperform-younger-foundersshattering-ageism/.

18. Patrick Button and David Neumark, "Age Discrimination's Challenge to the American Economy," NBER, October 11, 2022, https://www.nber.org/reporter/2022number3/age-discriminations-challenge-american-economy.

19. Ken Dychtwald, "How Innovative Employers Engage Older Workers—Part 1," LinkedIn, August 4, 2021, https://www.linkedin.com/pulse/how-innovative-employers-engage-older-workers-part-1-ken-dychtwald/.

20. Diana Kachan et al., "Health Status of Older US Workers and Nonworkers, National Health Interview Survey, 1997–2011," *Preventing Chronic Disease* 12 (September 24, 2015), https://doi.org/10.5888/pcd12.150040.

21. Chenkai Wu et al., "Association of Retirement Age with Mortality: A Population-Based Longitudinal Study Among Older Adults in the USA," *Journal of Epidemiology and Community Health* 70, no. 9 (March 21, 2016): 917–923, https://doi.org/10.1136/jech-2015-207097.

22. "Work It Boomers: Delaying Retirement May Slow Cognitive Decline," Psychiatrist.com, January 11, 2023, https://www.psychiatrist.com/news/work-it-boomers-delaying-retirement-may-slow-cognitive-decline/#:~:text=field%20were%20incomplete.-,Work%20It%20Boomers:%20Delaying%20Retirement%20May%20Slow%20Cognitive%20Decline,old%20age%2C%20the%20researchers%20speculated.

23. Anna Sundström, Michael Rönnlund, and Maria Josefsson, "A Nationwide Swedish Study of Age at Retirement and Dementia Risk," *International Journal of Geriatric Psychiatry* 35, no. 10 (June 19, 2020): 1243–1249, https://doi.org/10.1002/gps.5363.

24. Dana Wilkie, "What's the Difference Between a 'Good' Job and a 'Bad' Job?," SHRM, December 21, 2023, https://www.shrm.org/topics-tools/news/employee-relations/whats-difference-good-job-bad-job.

25. Mika Kivimäki et al., "Cognitive Stimulation in the Workplace, Plasma Proteins, and Risk of Dementia: Three Analyses of Population Cohort Studies," *BMJ*, August 19, 2021, n1804, https://doi.org/10.1136/bmj.n1804.

26. Philipp Hessel, "Does Retirement (Really) Lead to Worse Health Among European Men and Women Across All Educational Levels?," *Social Science and Medicine* 151 (February 2016): 19–26, https://doi.org/10.1016/j.socscimed.2015.12.018.

27. Takao Suzuki et al., "Are Japanese Older Adults Rejuvenating? Changes in Health-Related Measures Among Older Community Dwellers in the Last Decade," *Rejuvenation Research* 24, no. 1 (February 15, 2021): 37–48, https://doi.org/10.1089/rej.2019.2291.

28. Tetsuhiro Kidokoro et al., "Walking Speed and Balance Both Improved in Older Japanese Adults Between 1998 and 2018," *Journal of Exercise Science and Fitness* 19, no. 3 (July 2021): 204–208, https://doi.org/10.1016/j.jesf.2021.06.001.

29. Suzuki et al., "Are Japanese Older Adults Rejuvenating? Changes in Health-Related Measures Among Older Community Dwellers in the Last Decade."

30. Not surprisingly, advances in the physical capacity of older adults have been felt less strongly in the US, the UK, and other Western countries. Researchers have found that the advances in healthy life expectancy in the UK have not kept pace with advances in overall life expectancy. For instance, between 1996 and 2014, life expectancy at age fifty rose by 4.1 years for women in the UK, while healthy life expectancy increased by only 1.91 years during the same period. John W. Rowe and Lisa Berkman, "Decompression of Morbidity and the Workforce," *Nature Aging* 2 (January 20, 2022): 3–4, https://doi.org/10.1038/s43587-021-00163-y. The goal should be to get to a "compression of morbidity"—longer lives and fewer years in poor health—and instead we are getting something a little different: more years in good health and more years in poor health. It's an important fact to note about the UK, but it fundamentally still means that we are adding healthy years to life—just not as many as we might hope given life expectancy advances.

31. "Muscle Suit," Innophys, n.d., https://innophys.net/musclesuit/.

32. "A Third of Japanese People Aged 70 to 74 Still in the Workforce," nippon.com, October 10, 2023, https://www.nippon.com/en/japan-data/h01797/.

33. Lee Yeon-Woo, "Where Did All the Young Taxi Drivers Go?," *The Korea Times*, October 12, 2022, https://www.koreatimes.co.kr/www/nation/2024/11/113_337693.html.

34. Ivan Png, "Commentary: It's Worth Rethinking the Role of Taxis in Our Transport Network, as Industry Shrinks," *Channel News Asia*, September 9, 2024, https://www.channelnewsasia.com/commentary/singapore-no-taxi-grab-ride-hail-transport-4592636#:~:text=By%20statute%2C%20taxi%20drivers%20must,with%20the%20passage%20of%20time.

35. Gearoid Reidy, "Commentary: Wanted—80-year-old Taxi Drivers to Ease Japan's Labour Crunch," *Channel News Asia*, October 26, 2023, https://www.channel newsasia.com/commentary/japan-ageing-population-labour-crunch-old-taxi-drivers -3871431.

36. Xiao Lin et al., "Effects of Aging on Taxi Service Performance: A Comparative Study Based on Different Age Groups," *Sustainability* 15, no. 22 (November 20, 2023): 16096, https://doi.org/10.3390/su152216096.

37. Kim Ah-Jin, "From a Corporate Executive to a Startup Intern; I'm Not Obsessed with My Past Self," *Chosun Daily*, November 18, 2023, https://www.chosun.com /national/weekend/2023/11/18/AG3EEQT2FJE5LA3PJWA6SRJKY4/.

38. Daniel A. Cox and Sam Pressler, "Disconnected: The Growing Class Divide in American Civic Life—the Survey Center on American Life," Survey Center on American Life, August 22, 2024, https://www.americansurveycenter.org/research/disconnected -places-and-spaces/.

39. Dean Baker, "The Decline of Blue-Collar Jobs, in Graphs," Center for Economic and Policy Research, February 22, 2017, https://www.cepr.net/the-decline -of-blue-collar-jobs-in-graphs/#:~:text=In%201970%2C%20blue%2Dcollar%20 jobs,the%20growth%20in%20total%20employment.

40. "Ageing," The World Health Organization, n.d., https://www.who.int/health -topics/ageing#tab=tab_1.

41. "The Ratio of Workers to Social Security Beneficiaries Is at a Low and Projected to Decline Further," Peter G. Peterson Foundation, August 4, 2022, https:// www.pgpf.org/blog/2022/08/the-ratio-of-workers-to-social-security-beneficiaries -is-at-a-low-and-projected-to-decline-further#:~:text=A%20major%20contributor %20to%20the,exceeding%20revenues%20($1%2C088%20billion).

42. "Longevity Economy Principles: The Foundation for a Financially Resilient Future," World Economic Forum, January 2024, https://www3.weforum.org/docs/WEF _Longevity_Economy_Principles_2024.pdf. I served on the World Economic Forum Steering Committee for this report.

43. "Average Retirement Age for Men and Women, 1962–2016," Center for Retirement Research at Boston College, n.d., https://crr.bc.edu/wp-content/uploads/2021/03 /Average-retirement-age_2017-CPS.pdf.

44. Teresa Ghilarducci, "America Needs to Improve How It Treats Its Older Workers," *Forbes*, January 28, 2023, https://www.forbes.com/sites/teresaghilarducci /2023/01/28/how-america-treats-its-older-workers-new-data/.

45. "How Employers and Recruiters Are Overlooking the Talents of Over 50s Workers," Centre for Ageing Better, n.d., https://www.employment-studies.co.uk/system /files/resources/files/Shut-out-how-employers-and-recruiters-overlooking-talents -older-workers.pdf?_sm_nck=1.

46. Esme Fuller-Thomson, Jason Ferreirinha, and Katherine Marie Ahlin, "Temporal Trends (from 2008 to 2017) in Functional Limitations and Limitations in Activities of Daily Living: Findings from a Nationally Representative Sample of 5.4 Million Older Americans," *International Journal of Environmental Research and Public Health* 20, no. 3 (February 2, 2023): 2665, https://doi.org/10.3390/ijerph20032665.

47. Richard Fry and Dana Braga, "1. The Growth of the Older Workforce," Pew Research Center, December 14, 2023, https://www.pewresearch.org/social-trends/2023/12/14/the-growth-of-the-older-workforce/#:~:text=Among%20them:,workers%20did%20in%20the%20past.

48. Fry and Braga, "1. The Growth of the Older Workforce."

49. Erica Pandey, "Work Friendships Fade in Remote Era," Axios, June 2, 2024, https://www.axios.com/2024/06/02/work-friends-remote-hybrid-workplace-loneliness.

50. Constance Noonan Hadley and Sarah L. Wright, "We're Still Lonely at Work," Harvard Business Review, November 2024, https://hbr.org/2024/11/were-still-lonely-at-work. Hadley and Wright point out that while remote workers are more lonely than in-person workers, there are many factors other than work geography that impact loneliness and satisfaction among workers. Simply bringing people back to the office will not alone solve worker loneliness and depression.

51. E. S. Kim et al., "United We Thrive: Friendship and Subsequent Physical, Behavioural and Psychosocial Health in Older Adults (an Outcome-Wide Longitudinal Approach)," Epidemiology and Psychiatric Sciences 32 (November 15, 2023), https://doi.org/10.1017/s204579602300077x.

52. "47 Entreprises Sont Désormais Signataires De La Charte En Faveur De L'emploi Des +50 Ans," Club Landoy, April 7, 2023, https://www.clublandoy.com/47-entreprises-sont-desormais-signataires-de-la-charte-en-faveur-de-lemploi-des-50-ans/.

53. Linda Childers, "More Older Workers Are Applying for Entry-Level Jobs, Survey Finds," AARP, October 26, 2023, https://www.aarp.org/work/careers/older-workers-entry-level-jobs/.

Chapter 3: All Mixed Up

1. "Institution and Projects," Fundación Amancio Ortega, n.d., https://www.faortega.org/en/. And not by a small amount. Ortega's wealth has been estimated at over $100 billion, more than ten times the wealth of the next richest person in Spain at the time of this writing. "Forbes Real Time Billionaires List: The World's Richest People," Forbes, n.d., https://www.forbes.com/real-time-billionaires/#735d42973d78.

2. Marc Freedman, How to Live Forever: The Enduring Power of Connecting the Generations (PublicAffairs, 2018).

3. Carrianne J. Leschak and Naomi I. Eisenberger, "Two Distinct Immune Pathways Linking Social Relationships with Health: Inflammatory and Antiviral Processes," Psychosomatic Medicine 81, no. 8 (October 2019): 711–719, https://doi.org/10.1097/psy.0000000000000685.

4. Tian Q, "Intergeneration Social Support Affects the Subjective Well-Being of the Elderly: Mediator Roles of Self-Esteem and Loneliness," Journal of Health Psychology 21, no. 6 (2016): 1137–1144.

Alejandro Canedo-García et al., "Evaluation of the Benefits, Satisfaction, and Limitations of Intergenerational Face-to-Face Activities: A General Population Survey in Spain," International Journal of Environmental Research and Public Health 18, no. 18 (September 14, 2021): 9683, https://doi.org/10.3390/ijerph18189683. Anna Krzeczkowska, David M. Spalding, William J. McGeown, Alan J. Gow, Michelle C. Carlson, and Louise A. Brown Nicholls, "A Systematic Review of the Impacts of Intergenerational Engagement on Older Adults' Cognitive, Social, and Health Outcomes," *Ageing Research Reviews* 71 (2021): 101400, https://www.sciencedirect.com/science/article/pii /S1568163721001471?via%3Dihub.

5. Daniel W. L. Lai et al., "The Impact of Intergenerational Relationship on Health and Well-Being of Older Chinese Americans," *Journal of the American Geriatrics Society* 67, no. S3 (August 12, 2019), https://doi.org/10.1111/jgs.15893.

6. John M. Ruiz, Patrick Steffen, and Timothy B. Smith, "Hispanic Mortality Paradox: A Systematic Review and Meta-Analysis of the Longitudinal Literature," *American Journal of Public Health* 103, no. 3 (February 6, 2013): e52–60, https://doi .org/10.2105/ajph.2012.301103.

7. Lai et al., "The Impact of Intergenerational Relationship on Health and Well-Being of Older Chinese Americans," August 12, 2019.

8. William H. Frey, "Neighborhood Segregation Persists for Black, Latino or Hispanic, and Asian Americans," Brookings, April 6, 2021, https://www.brookings .edu/articles/neighborhood-segregation-persists-for-black-latino-or-hispanic-and -asian-americans/#:~:text=At%20the%20same%20time%2C%20Black,variations %20in%20these%20segregation%20patterns.

9. Christina A. Samuels, "Segregation of Latino Students from White Peers Increased over a Generation, Study Finds," *Education Week*, July 30, 2019, https://www .edweek.org/leadership/segregation-of-latino-students-from-white-peers-increased -over-a-generation-study-finds/2019/07.

10. Richelle Winkler, "Research Note: Segregated by Age: Are We Becoming More Divided?," *Population Research and Policy Review* 32, no. 4 (July 11, 2013): 717–727, https://doi.org/10.1007/s11113-013-9291-8.

11. Marc Freedman and Trent Stamp, "The U.S. Isn't Just Getting Older. It's Getting More Segregated by Age," *Harvard Business Review*, June 6, 2018, https://hbr.org /2018/06/the-u-s-isnt-just-getting-older-its-getting-more-segregated-by-age#:~:text =%E2%80%9CI%20think%20we're%20in,without%20contact%20with%20older%20 people. Quoting Cornell Professor Karl Pillemer.

12. For a general read on Del Webb, see Margaret Finnerty and Tara Blanc, *Del Webb: A Man, a Company* (Heritage Publishers, 1998). Freedman's *How to Live Forever* has a more specific recounting of the origins of Sun City.

13. Eileen Daspin, "Niche Retirement Communities Are Growing—Are They Right for You?," Kiplinger.com, April 25, 2024, https://www.kiplinger.com/retirement/niche -retirement-communities-are-growing-are-they-right-for-you.

14. Freedman, *How to Live Forever*, 103.

15. "Family Matters: Multigenerational Living Is on the Rise and Here to Stay," Generations United, 2021, https://www.gu.org/app/uploads/2021/04/21-MG-Family -Report-WEB.pdf.

16. "All in Together," Generations United and the Eisner Foundation, 2018, https://www.gu.org/resources/all-in-together-creating-places-where-young-and-old-thrive/.

17. "Tree Conservation," National Parks Board, n.d., https://www.nparks.gov.sg/treessg/learn/tree-conservation.

18. "Pilot Health District in Queenstown to Focus on Residents' Holistic Well-Being," National University of Singapore, October 20, 2021, https://news.nus.edu.sg/pilot-health-district-in-queenstown-to-focus-on-residents-holistic-well-being/.

19. "How We Get Around," Barcelona Metropolis, September 2021, https://www.barcelona.cat/metropolis/en/contents/how-we-get-around#:~:text=Barcelona%20Metropolis&text=Laura%20Navarro%20is%20a%20data%20journalist.&text=Barcelona%20tops%20the%20list%20of,accidents%20is%20becoming%20increasingly%20significant.

20. Pablo Valerio, "Barcelona's First Superblock, Fighting the Power of Habit and Wavering Political Will," Cities of the Future, October 13, 2016, https://citiesofthefuture.eu/barcelonas-first-superblock-fighting-the-power-of-habit-and-wavering-political-will/.

21. William Tsang, Gloria Wong, and Kelly Gao, "Mahjong Playing and Eye-Hand Coordination in Older Adults—a Cross-Sectional Study," *Journal of Physical Therapy Science* 28, no. 10 (October 2016), 2955–2960, https://www.jstage.jst.go.jp/article/jpts/28/10/28_jpts-2016-573/_article.

22. Jason Horowitz, "The Lost Days That Made Bergamo a Coronavirus Tragedy," *New York Times*, February 2, 2021, https://www.nytimes.com/2020/11/29/world/europe/coronavirus-bergamo-italy.html.

23. "Playful Paradigm Makes the Healthy Choice the Enjoyable Choice," URBACT, February 6, 2017, https://urbact.eu/good-practices/playful-paradigm-makes-healthy-choice-enjoyable-choice.

24. Joe Verghese et al., "Leisure Activities and the Risk of Dementia in the Elderly," *New England Journal of Medicine* 348, no. 25 (June 19, 2003): 2508–2516, https://doi.org/10.1056/nejmoa022252.

25. Ashton Applewhite, *This Chair Rocks: A Manifesto Against Ageism* (Networked Books, Inc., 2016), 185–188.

26. Applewhite, *This Chair Rocks*, 187.

27. Donna Butts, "Family Matters: Multigenerational Living Is on the Rise and Here to Stay," 2021.

28. Dipo Fadeyi and Juliana Menasce Horowitz, "Americans More Likely to Say It's a Bad Thing than a Good Thing That More Young Adults Live with Their Parents," Pew Research Center, https://www.pewresearch.org/short-reads/2022/08/24/americans-more-likely-to-say-its-a-bad-thing-than-a-good-thing-that-more-young-adults-live-with-their-parents/.

29. Ashley Powdar, "How the Employer Pledge Program Helps Older Workers Get Hired," AARP, September 9, 2022, https://www.aarp.org/work/job-search/employer-pledge-program-helps-older-workers/.

Chapter 4: *The Tomato, the Asparagus, and the Carrot*

1. "Around the Globe, Women Outlive Men," PRB, September 1, 2001, https://www.prb.org/resources/around-the-globe-women-outlive-men/.

2. Ani Petrosyan, "Daily Time Spent Online by Users Worldwide Q2 2024, by Region," Statista, November 5, 2024, https://www.statista.com/statistics/1258232/daily-time-spent-online-worldwide/.

3. Erika Spissu, Naveen Eluru, Ram M. Pendyala, and Karthik Konduri, "A Comparative Analysis of Weekday Time Use and Activity Patterns Between Italy and the United States," University of Texas, n.d., https://www.caee.utexas.edu/prof/bhat/abstracts/italy_us_timeusecomparison_1aug07.pdf.

4. "Study on Volunteering in the European Union: Country Report Italy," European Volunteer Centre, 2006, https://ec.europa.eu/citizenship/pdf/national_report_it_en.pdf.

5. "Countries with Highest Numbers of Volunteers: USA, Canada, Australia, UK, France, and Many More," Volunteer FDIP, January 5, 2025, https://www.volunteerfdip.org/countries-with-highest-numbers-of-volunteers-usa-canada-australia-uk-france#google_vignette.

6. Gian Paolo Barbetta et al., "Entry and Exit of Nonprofit Organizations," *Nonprofit Policy Forum* 9, no. 2 (August 21, 2018), https://doi.org/10.1515/npf-2017-0036.

7. Lucia Boccacin, "Volunteering and Active Aging in Italy," *International Journal of Aging and Society* 7, no. 1 (2016): 77–90, https://staging-unicatt.elsevierpure.com/en/publications/volunteering-and-active-aging-in-italy-8.

8. Barbetta et al., "Entry and Exit of Nonprofit Organizations," August 21, 2018.

9. Lars Olov Bygren et al., "Association Between Attending Cultural Events and All-Cause Mortality: A Longitudinal Study with Three Measurements (1982–2017)," *BMJ Open* 13, no. 2 (February 21, 2023): e065714, https://doi.org/10.1136/bmjopen-2022-065714.

10. Olov Bygren et al., "Association Between Attending Cultural Events and All-Cause Mortality," e065714.

11. Dietmar Ausserhofer et al., "Community-Dwelling Older Adults' Readiness for Adopting Digital Health Technologies: Cross-Sectional Survey Study," *JMIR Formative Research* 8 (April 2024): e54120, https://pmc.ncbi.nlm.nih.gov/articles/PMC11094597/pdf/formative_v8i1e54120.pdf.

12. Justin Ladner, "How Older Adults Lead the Way in American Volunteerism," NationSwell, September 25, 2023, https://nationswell.com/older-adults-lead-the-way/#:~:text=Consequently%2C%20the%20share%20of%20total,19%20posed%20for%20older%20adults.

13. Linda P. Fried et al., "Experience Corps: A Dual Trial to Promote the Health of Older Adults and Children's Academic Success," *Contemporary Clinical Trials* 36, no. 1 (September 2013): 1–13, https://doi.org/10.1016/j.cct.2013.05.003.

14. "Press Release: Volunteering Reduces Risk of Hypertension in Older Adults, Carnegie Mellon Research Shows," Carnegie Mellon University, June 13, 2013, https://www.cmu.edu/news/stories/archives/2013/june/june13_volunteeringhypertension

.html#:~:text=New%20research%20from%20Carnegie%20Mellon,blood%20pressure %2C%20by%2040%20percent.

15. "2017 State of the Evidence Annual Report," Corporation for National and Community Service, 2017, https://americorps.gov/evidence-exchange/2017-state-evidence -annual-report.

16. Kasley Killam, *The Art and Science of Connection: Why Social Health Is the Missing Key to Living Longer, Healthier, and Happier* (HarperOne, 2024), 121.

17. Nancy Morrow-Howell et al., "Effects of Volunteering on the Well-Being of Older Adults," *The Journals of Gerontology Series B* 58, no. 3 (May 2003): S137–S145, https://doi.org/10.1093/geronb/58.3.s137.

18. "Volunteering and Civic Life in America," AmeriCorps, n.d., https://americorps .gov/about/our-impact/volunteering-civic-life#:~:text=Informal%20Helping%20The %20share%20of%20Americans%20who,of%203%20percentage%20points%20 over%20previous%20years.

19. Julia S. Nakamura et al., "Informal Helping and Subsequent Health and Well-Being in Older U.S. Adults," *International Journal of Behavioral Medicine* 31, no. 4 (May 26, 2023): 503–515, https://doi.org/10.1007/s12529-023-10187-w.

20. Laurie Vazquez, "The Secret to Living Past 100? Lots of Sex. Also, Rosemary.," Big Think, September 13, 2016, https://bigthink.com/culture-religion/the-secret-to -living-past-100-lots-of-sex-also-rosemary/.

21. Saul Justin Newman, "Supercentenarian and Remarkable Age Records Exhibit Patterns Indicative of Clerical Errors and Pension Fraud," *bioRxiv (Cold Spring Harbor Laboratory)*, March 14, 2024, https://www.biorxiv.org/content/10.1101/704080v3. Newman's research noted that few supercentenarians have validated birth certificates and that they tend to be clustered in areas with poor recordkeeping, low literacy rates, high poverty rates, and high crime rates. He also noted that the birthdates of super-centenarians in places like Okinawa are suspiciously concentrated on days divisible by five, suggestive of clerical errors or fraud. "'The Data on Extreme Human Ageing Is Rotten from the Inside Out'—Ig Nobel Winner Saul Justin Newman," The Conversation, September 13, 2024, https://theconversation.com/the-data-on-extreme-human -ageing-is-rotten-from-the-inside-out-ig-nobel-winner-saul-justin-newman-239023.

22. "List of Countries by Traffic-Related Death Rate," Wikipedia, accessed November 5, 2024, https://en.wikipedia.org/wiki/List_of_countries_by_traffic-related _death_rate.

23. Juliette Gagliargi, "Italy: Overweight and Obese Adults by Region 2023," Statista, April 30, 2024, https://www.statista.com/statistics/794633/overweight-and-obesity -among-adults-by-region-in-italy/#:~:text=In%202023%2C%20Apulia%20was%20 the,51%20and%2050%20percent%2C%20respectively.

24. Bianca Spaggiari, "Caffè Sospeso: The Neapolitan Tradition of Buying Coffee for Someone Who Can't," *Italy Segreta*, December 20, 2023, https://italysegreta.com /caffe-sospeso/.

25. Miya Chang, "Comparative Study on Volunteering Among Older Korean Immigrants in the United States and Older Koreans in South Korea," *International*

Journal of Environmental Research and Public Health 19, no. 12 (June 14, 2022): 7297, https://doi.org/10.3390/ijerph19127297.

26. Nathan Dietz and Robert T. Grimm Jr., "Understanding Generosity: A Look at What Influences Volunteering and Giving in the United States," Do Good Institute, November 2023, https://dogood.umd.edu/sites/default/files/2023-10/Understanding GenerosityReport_DoGoodInstitute_11.2023.pdf.

27. Joe Heim, "Nonprofits Need More Help than Ever: Why Aren't Americans Volunteering?," *Washington Post*, December 11, 2023, https://www.washingtonpost.com/dc-md-va/2023/12/09/volunteer-decline-homeless-pandemic/.

28. Harriet Whitehead, "Small Charities Hit Hardest by Volunteering Falling to Record Low, Say Researchers," May 21, 2024, https://www.civilsociety.co.uk/news/small-charities-hit-hardest-by-volunteering-falling-to-record-low-say-researchers.html#:~:text=PBE%20compared%20its%20findings%20to,27%25%20in%20 2013%2D14.

29. Ben Evans, "Present Struggles, Past Origins: Current Challenges in Volunteering Amidst Two Decades of Decline," VCSE Data and Insights National Observatory, May 2024, https://www.ntu.ac.uk/__data/assets/pdf_file/0027/2391840/VCSE-barometer-wave-6-report-may-2024.pdf.

30. "Germany: Web Starter Kit," AARP International, n.d., https://www.aarpinternational.org/initiatives/aging-readiness-competitiveness-arc/germany#:~:text=Innovative%20programs%20include%20shared%20living,connecting%20them%20 to%20volunteer%20opportunities.

31. Kathrin Komp, Kees Van Kersbergen, and Theo Van Tilburg, "Policies for Older Volunteers: A Study of Germany and Italy, 1990–2008," *Journal of Aging Studies* 27, no. 4 (December 2013): 443–455, https://doi.org/10.1016/j.jaging.2013.10.003.

32. Nancy Morrow-Howell, "Volunteering in Later Life: Research Frontiers," *The Journals of Gerontology: Series B* 65B, no. 4 (July 2010): 461–469, https://pubmed.ncbi.nlm.nih.gov/20400498/.

33. Rose Hoban, "Life Expectancy Gap Widens for Appalachia," *North Carolina Health News*, August 30, 2017, https://www.northcarolinahealthnews.org/2017/08/30/life-expectancy-gap-widens-appalachia/.

34. "Exploring Bright Spots in Appalachian Health: Case Studies," Appalachian Regional Commission, July 2018, https://arc.gov/wp-content/uploads/2020/06/BrightSpotsCaseStudiesJuly2018.pdf.

35. Aarefa Johari, "India Has 2 Million Non-Profits—and No, That's Not a Lot," *Quartz*, March 1, 2014, https://qz.com/182757/india-has-2-million-non-profits-and-thats-not-a-lot#:~:text=This%20week%2C%20India's%20Central%20Bureau,figure%20could%20be%20much%20higher.

36. Eric S. Kim, Ashley V. Whillans, Matthew T. Lee, Ying Chen, and Tyler J. VanderWeele, "Volunteering and Subsequent Health and Well-Being in Older Adults: An Outcome-Wide Longitudinal Approach," *American Journal of Preventive Medicine* 59, no. 2 (August 2020): 176–186, https://pubmed.ncbi.nlm.nih.gov/32536452/.

37. Eric Burger, "40 Volunteer Statistics That Will Blow Your Mind," *Volunteer Hub* (blog), November 9, 2021, https://volunteerhub.com/blog/40-volunteer-statistics #:~:text=4%25%20of%20college%20graduates%2C%2025,only%20one%20organization %20each%20year.

38. Victoria Catterall-Decalmer, "How Much Time Do Americans Spend on Their Health and Fitness?," MyProtein, 2019, https://us.myprotein.com/thezone/training /american-health-fitness-survey/.

39. Amy Yotopoulos, "Three Reasons Why People Don't Volunteer, and What Can Be Done About It," Stanford Center on Longevity, n.d., https://longevity.stanford .edu/three-reasons-why-people-dont-volunteer-and-what-can-be-done-about-it/.

40. Nancy Galambos, Harvey Krahn, Matthew Johnson, and Marjorie Lachman, "The U Shape of Happiness Across the Life Course: Expanding the Discussion," *Perspectives on Psychological Science* 15, no. 4 (May 6, 2020): 898–912, https://pmc .ncbi.nlm.nih.gov/articles/PMC7529452/.

Chapter 5: *The Last Acceptable "Ism"*

1. Mathew Mathews and Paulin Tay Straughan, "Results from the Perception and Attitudes Towards Ageing and Seniors Survey (2013/2014)," Singapore Management University, October 2014, https://ink.library.smu.edu.sg/cgi/viewcontent.cgi?article =3477&context=soss_research.

2. Reuben Ng, Nicole Indran, and Luyao Liu, "Social Media Discourse on Ageism, Sexism, and Racism: Analysis of 150 Million Tweets over 15 Years," *Journal of the American Geriatrics Society* 72, no. 10 (July 3, 2024), https://doi.org/10.1111jgs.19047.

3. "The Heart of Care," Agency for Integrated Care, https://www.aic.sg/the-heart -of-care/.

4. Boo Ping Er, "The Agency for Integrated Care Takes on 'Ok Boomer' Saying in New Campaign," *Marketing-Interactive*, January 15, 2024, https://www.marketing -interactive.com/aic-break-the-silver-ceiling-ok-boomer.

5. Becca Levy, *Breaking the Age Code: How Your Beliefs About Aging Determine How Long and Well You Live* (William Morrow, 2022), 105.

6. Lisa Wallin, "Japanese Holidays: What Is 'Keiro No Hi' (Respect for the Aged Day)?," *Tokyo Weekender*, September 18, 2021, https://www.tokyoweekender.com /art_and_culture/japanese-culture/japanese-holidays-what-is-keiro-no-hi-respect -for-the-aged-day/. Keiro no Hi was first celebrated in Taka town in Hyogo Prefecture in 1947 in the hopes that it would encourage young people to support older residents after the hardships of World War II. Called Elderly People's Day, the holiday celebrated people fifty-five and older. Times change, as has the name of the holiday and the definition of aged. There is no specific age cutoff for who gets feted and who doesn't, but not surprisingly in a country with more than 36 million people over the age of sixty-five (almost 30 percent of the population), fifty-five-year-olds no longer get celebrated. Typically, people have to be seventy or older to qualify as celebrants now, and that threshold is likely to climb higher in the future.

7. Motoko Rich, "A Woman Who Shows Age Is No Barrier to Talk Show Stardom," *New York Times*, January 19, 2024, https://www.nytimes.com/2024/01/19/world/asia /tetsuko-kuroyanagi-japan-television.html.

8. Levy, *Breaking the Age Code*, 4.

9. Levy, *Breaking the Age Code*, 113.

10. Becca R. Levy, Martin D. Slade, E-Shien Chang, Sneha Kannoth, and Shi-Yi Wang, "Ageism Amplifies Cost and Prevalence of Health Conditions," *The Gerontologist* 60, no. 1 (February 2020): 174–181, https://academic.oup.com/gerontologist/article /60/1/174/5166947.

11. B. R. Levy and M. D. Slade, "Role of Positive Age Beliefs in Recovery from Mild Cognitive Impairment Among Older Persons," *JAMA Network Open* 6, no. 4 (April 12, 2023): e237707, https://jamanetwork.com/journals/jamanetworkopen/full article/2803740.

12. B. Levy and E. Langer, "Aging Free from Negative Stereotypes: Successful Memory in China Among the American Deaf," *Journal of Personality and Social Psychology* 66, no. 6 (1994): 989–997, https://doi.org/10.1037/0022-3514.66.6.989.

13. Applewhite, *This Chair Rocks: A Manifesto Against Ageism*, 6.

14. Bess Levin, "Texas Lt. Governor: Old People Should Volunteer to Die to Save the Economy," *Vanity Fair*, March 24, 2020, https://www.vanityfair.com/news/2020/03 /dan-patrick-coronavirus-grandparents?srsltid=AfmBOopfU-i8nzI6JZtPqWIvp Ad6bMKyvuFh5HEyPE-X-kTYSeKgcvND.

15. "The Physician Shortage in Geriatrics," ChenMed, March 18, 2022, https:// www.chenmed.com/blog/physician-shortage-geriatrics.

16. Reuben Ng and Jeremy W. Lim-Soh, "Ageism Linked to Culture, Not Demographics: Evidence from an 8-Billion-Word Corpus Across 20 Countries," *The Journals of Gerontology: Series B* 76, no. 9 (November 2021): 1791–1798, https://doi .org/10.1093/geronb/gbaa181.

17. Sui-Lee Wee, "Why Southeast Asia Is Crying over This Movie," *New York Times*, June 23, 2024, https://www.nytimes.com/2024/06/23/world/asia/make-millions -before-grandma-dies-crying.html.

18. Raphael Rashid, "'Fashion Has No Age': The Stylish Senior Citizens of Seoul," *The Guardian*, May 12, 2022, https://www.theguardian.com/world/2022/may/12/kim -dong-hyun-seoul-stylish-senior-citizens.

19. Naomi Chadderton, "Breaking Age Barriers: How Fashion Week Is Embracing Mature Female Models," Life/Redefined, n.d., https://life-redefined.co/lifestyle /fashion-week#:~:text=From%20an%20increasing%20number%20of,a%20 life%2C%E2%80%9D%20he%20added.

20. Elizabeth Paton, "Age Is Not a Problem," *New York Times*, March 12, 2024, https://www.nytimes.com/2024/03/12/style/models-fashion-age.html.

21. Reuben Ng and Nicole Indran, "Hostility Toward Baby Boomers on TikTok," *The Gerontologist* 62, no. 8 (February 1, 2022): 1196–1206, https://doi.org/10.1093 /geront/gnac020.

22. W. J. Nusselder et al., "Women's Excess Unhealthy Life Years: Disentangling the Unhealthy Life Years Gap," *European Journal of Public Health* 29, no. 5 (July 5, 2019): 914–919, https://academic.oup.com/eurpub/article/29/5/914/5529190.

23. Patwardhan Vedavati et al., "Differences Across the Lifespan Between Females and Males in the Top 20 Causes of Disease Burden Globally: A Systematic Analysis of the Global Burden of Disease Study 2021," *The Lancet Public Health* 9, no. 5 (May 2024): e282–e294, https://www.thelancet.com/journals/lanpub/article/PIIS2468-2667(24)00053-7/fulltext.

24. Ayaka Kibi, "Average Life Expectancy in Japan Up for 1st Time in 3 Years," *The Asahi Shimbun*, July 27, 2024, https://www.asahi.com/ajw/articles/15364723#:~:text=For%20men%2C%20the%20figure%20was,%2C%20%E2%80%9D%20said%20a%20ministry%20official.&text=Compiled%20from%20Ministry%20of%20Health,countries%20use%20different%20statistical%20methods.

25. Mayumi Karasawa et al., "Cultural Perspectives on Aging and Well-Being: A Comparison of Japan and the U.S.," *International Journal of Aging and Human Development* 73, no. 1 (July 29, 2011): 73–98, https://journals.sagepub.com/doi/10.2190/AG.73.1.d.

Chapter 6: *Wrinkles in Time: Building the Social Superhighway*

1. Chelsea Strub, "Study Shows High Cancer Rates in Northeast Pennsylvania," *WNEP News*, January 18, 2023, https://www.wnep.com/article/news/local/lackawanna-county/new-study-shows-high-cancer-rates-northeast-regional-cancer-institute-pennsylvania/523-64808b9a-b5e1-4e3a-b357-495a5288f533.

2. Nina Goldman et al., "Addressing Loneliness and Social Isolation in 52 Countries: A Scoping Review of National Policies," *BMC Public Health* 24, no. 1 (May 1, 2024), https://doi.org/10.1186/s12889-024-18370-8.

3. "Murphy: The Right and Left Can Come Together to Address the Epidemic of Loneliness," Chris Murphy, June 22, 2023, https://www.murphy.senate.gov/newsroom/press-releases/murphy-the-right-and-left-can-come-together-to-address-the-epidemic-of-loneliness.

4. Killam, *The Art and Science of Connection*, 15.

5. Nicholas Epley and Juliana Schroeder, "Mistakenly Seeking Solitude," *Journal of Experimental Psychology: General* 143, no. 5 (July 4, 2014), https://psycnet.apa.org/record/2014-28833-001.

6. Phil Edwards, "When Running for Exercise Was for Weirdos," *Vox*, August 9, 2015, https://www.vox.com/2015/8/9/9115981/running-jogging-history.

7. Andrew K. Yegian, Steven B. Heymsfield, Daniel E. Lieberman, "Historical Body Temperature Records as a Population-Level 'Thermometer' of Physical Activity in the United States," *Current Biology* 31, no. 20 (October 25, 2021): R1375–R1376, https://www.cell.com/current-biology/fulltext/S0960-9822(21)01254-9?_returnURL=https%3A%2F%2Flinkinghub.elsevier.com%2Fretrieve%2Fpii%2FS0960982221012549%3Fshowall%3Dtrue.

8. Annemarie H. Sammartino, *Freedomland: Co-op City and the Story of New York* (Three Hills, 2022).

9. Jeffrey M. Jones, "Church Attendance Has Declined in Most U.S. Religious Groups," Gallup, March 25, 2024, https://news.gallup.com/poll/642548/church-attendance-declined-religious-groups.aspx#:~:text=Two%20decades%20ago%2C%20an%20average,do%20not%20attend%20services%20regularly. Greg Rosalsky, "You May Have Heard of the 'Union Boom.' The Numbers Tell a Different Story," *NPR*, February 28, 2023, https://www.npr.org/sections/money/2023/02/28/1159663461/you-may-have-heard-of-the-union-boom-the-numbers-tell-a-different-story.

10. Matthew McGough et al., "How Do Health Expenditures Vary Across the Population?," Peterson-KFF Health System Tracker, January 4, 2024, https://www.healthsystemtracker.org/chart-collection/health-expenditures-vary-across-population/#Share%20of%20total%20population%20and%20total%20health%20spending,%20by%20age%20group,%202021.

11. Jonathan Lambert, "Living Near Your Grandmother Has Evolutionary Benefits," *NPR*, February 7, 2019, https://www.npr.org/sections/goatsandsoda/2019/02/07/692088371/living-near-your-grandmother-has-evolutionary-benefits#:~:text=In%20the%201960s%2C%20researchers%20came,grandchildren%20carrying%20their%20longevity%20genes.

12. Mark Nieuwenhuijsen et al., "The Superblock Model: A Review of an Innovative Urban Model for Sustainability, Liveability, Health and Well-Being," *Environmental Research* 251, no. 1 (June 15, 2024): 118550, https://www.sciencedirect.com/science/article/pii/S0013935124004547.

13. "Largest Year-to-Year Increase in Over 20 Years for Public School Spending per Pupil," US Census Bureau, April 25, 2024, https://www.census.gov/newsroom/press-releases/2024/public-school-spending-per-pupil.html#:~:text=Expenditures,up%20$84.2%20billion%20(9.8%25).

14. Annie Waldman, Aliyya Swaby, and Anna Clark, "America's Adult Education System Is Broken. Here's How Experts Say We Can Fix It.," *ProPublica*, December 23, 2022, https://www.propublica.org/article/literacy-adult-education-united-states-solutions#:~:text=The%20federal%20government%20provided%20about,not%20all%20adult%20education%20teachers.

15. Alice Milivinti and David Rehkopf, "A New Map of Life: Work," Stanford Center on Longevity, May 24, 2021, https://longevity.stanford.edu/wp-content/uploads/2021/11/Milivinti-Work-Report.pdf.

16. Viji Diane Kannan and Peter J. Veazie, "US Trends in Social Isolation, Social Engagement, and Companionship—Nationally and by Age, Sex, Race/Ethnicity, Family Income, and Work Hours, 2003–2020," *SSM—Population Health* 21 (2023): 101331, https://www.sciencedirect.com/science/article/pii/S235282732200310X?via%3Dihub.

17. In the United States, proposals to establish a national service platform for seniors have been floated from time to time; most recently, the writer Daniel Pink proposed putting the AmeriCorps Seniors program on financial steroids and getting America's seniors back to work. Daniel Pink, "Why Not Enlist an Army of Volunteer

Retirees?," *The Washington Post*, December 2, 2024, https://www.washingtonpost
.com/opinions/2024/12/02/seniors-service-americorps/. These are smart ideas which
could have significant health benefits to both communities and volunteers if ever
implemented. Sadly, that seems unlikely in the current political environment.

18. H. H. Fung and L. L. Carstensen, "Sending Memorable Messages to the Old:
Age Differences in Preferences and Memory for Advertisements," *Journal of Personality and Social Psychology* 85, no. 1 (July 2003): 163–178, https://psycnet.apa.org/record
/2003-05568-016.

INDEX

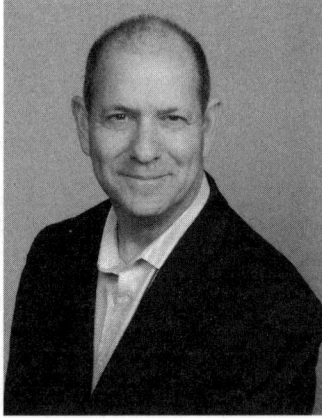

Ken Stern is a nationally recognized expert on longevity and aging. He is the founder of the Longevity Project and hosts the award-winning *Century Lives* podcast from the Stanford Center on Longevity. Stern is the author of *With Charity for All* and the national bestseller *Republican Like Me.* He has been a frequent contributor to a wide variety of publications, including *Vanity Fair, The Atlantic,* and *Slate.* He is also the former CEO of NPR. He lives in Washington, DC, with his wife, Beth, and son, Nate.

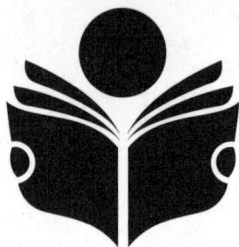

RAISING READERS
Books Build Bright Futures

Thank you for reading this book and for being a reader of books in general. A author, I am so grateful to share being part of a community of readers with and I hope you will join me in passing our love of books on to the next genera of readers.

Did you know that reading for enjoyment is the single biggest predictor child's future happiness and success?

More than family circumstances, parents' educational background, or inco reading impacts a child's future academic performance, emotional well-be communication skills, economic security, ambition, and happiness.

Studies show that kids reading for enjoyment in the US is in rapid decline:

- In 2012, 53% of 9-year-olds read almost every day. Just 10 years later, in 2022, the number had fallen to 39%.
- In 2012, 27% of 13-year-olds read for fun daily. By 2023, that number was just 14%.

Together, we can commit to **Raising Readers** and change this trend. How?

- Read to children in your life daily.
- Model reading as a fun activity.
- Reduce screen time.
- Start a family, school, or community book club.
- Visit bookstores and libraries regularly.
- Listen to audiobooks.
- Read the book before you see the movie.
- Encourage your child to read aloud to a pet or stuffed animal.
- Give books as gifts.
- Donate books to families and communities in need.

Books build bright futures, and **Raising Readers** is our shared responsibility

For more information, visit **JoinRaisingReaders.com**

Sources: National Endowment for the Arts, National Assessment of Educational Progress, WorldBookDay.org, Nielsen BookData's 2023 "Understanding the Children's Book Consumer"